PANORAMA OF THE PANDEMIC

This volume provides a multi-nuanced analysis of the impact of the Covid-19 pandemic on various aspects of human existence, encompassing societal, economic, and inter-relational dimensions. It highlights a broad range of artistic and literary experiences that unfolded as a consequence of the pandemic or speak to that time.

The book revisits pandemic-induced shifts, phenomenologically, including the digitization of art and representations of creativity, "performance" anxiety, socio-political climate determined by "racial algorithms," gaming surges, employment insecurities, mental health issues from a pedagogical materiality, and the nature of apocalypse through literary reimaginations. It also delves into the global food crisis, reframing of family structures, and local subjectivities as lived experiences.

A unique contribution, the book will be useful for students and researchers of cultural studies, digital humanities, mass media, sociology, mental health, psychology, medical anthropology, public health, literature, history of pandemics and epidemics, and South Asian studies.

Simi Malhotra is Professor, Department of English, Jamia Millia Islamia, Delhi, India.

Ruchi Nagpal has earned her doctoral degree from the Department of English, Jamia Millia Islamia, Delhi, India.

Steven S. George is a Ph.D. scholar at the Department of English, Jamia Millia Islamia, Delhi, India.

Sananda Roy has earned her doctoral degree from the Department of English, Jamia Millia Islamia, Delhi, India.

Academics, Politics and Society in the Post-COVID World

Series Editors: **Lewis Gordon**, Professor, University of Connecticut, USA; **Rozena Maart**, Professor, University of KwaZulu Natal, South Africa; **Epifania Amoo-Adare**, Independent Researcher, UK and Ghana; and **Sayan Dey**, Postdoctoral Fellow, University of Witwatersrand, South Africa.

This book series focuses on various forms of academic, social and political transformations that are taking place/are expected to take place in a post-COVID World. The biomedical crisis of COVID-19 has opened up a floodgate for all kinds of crisis like communal violence, racial discrimination, geographical hierarchies, socio-political hegemonies, and academic exclusivities. These crises are also catalyzing massive geo-political shifts in various epistemological and ontological frameworks of knowledge production across the globe. These shifts in turn are bound to influence patterns of thinking and doing in a post-COVID era, including shifts affecting pedagogical frameworks, curricular structures, institutional infrastructures, evaluation patterns, international policies, political ethics, communal relations, gender existence, racial connotations, mental health and physical wellbeing. With respect to academic shifts, many elite academic institutions have transferred their courses online, while other institutions are forced to shut down, due to the lack of sufficient technological infrastructure. With respect to politics, countries are experiencing several shifts in terms of social, cultural, economic and political policy-making that are bound to bring major changes in internal as well as international relations. With respect to society, the global pandemic has aggravated already existing racial, communal and cultural differences. At the same time, there are consistent efforts towards new forms of solidarities, reconciliations and humanity. All these are transformations that will continue to take place in a post-COVID era. Keeping these shifting scenarios at the forefront, this book series critically analyzes the various forms of transformation taking place in academic, social and political systems across the globe, during this post-COVID era.

Pandemic Fissures
COVID-19, Dehumanisation, and the Obsolescence of Freedom in India
Suddhabrata Deb Roy

Panorama of the Pandemic
A Phenomenological Inquiry
Simi Malhotra, Ruchi Nagpal, Steven S. George and Sananda Roy

PANORAMA OF THE PANDEMIC

A Phenomenological Inquiry

Edited by Simi Malhotra, Ruchi Nagpal, Steven S. George and Sananda Roy

Routledge
Taylor & Francis Group
LONDON AND NEW YORK

Designed cover image: Getty Images

First published 2025
by Routledge
4 Park Square, Milton Park, Abingdon, Oxon OX14 4RN

and by Routledge
605 Third Avenue, New York, NY 10158

Routledge is an imprint of the Taylor & Francis Group, an informa business

British Library Cataloguing-in-Publication Data
A catalogue record for this book is available from the British Library

ISBN: 978-1-032-90163-3 (hbk)
ISBN: 978-1-032-96673-1 (pbk)
ISBN: 978-1-003-59039-2 (ebk)

DOI: 10.4324/9781003590392

Typeset in Sabon
by SPi Technologies India Pvt Ltd (Straive)

CONTENTS

FIGURES

EDITORS

Steven S. George is a Ph.D. scholar at the Department of English, Jamia Millia Islamia. He was Visiting Scholar at the University of Witwatersrand (2021–2022) working with Prof. Dilip Menon on *Cosmopolitan Cultures and Oceanic Thought: Thinking through History across the Waters*. He was a Summer Fellow at Michigan State University (2022), working with Prof. Sean Pue on Digital Humanities, and received the Research Fellowship Award (2023) from the Christian Institute for the Study of Religion and Society. He has authored "Singing Rivers: Spatial Discourses and Milieu-Specific Analysis" in *Globalization and Sense-Making Practices*, published by Routledge (2023), and "Christianity, Conversion, and Caste" in *Cosmopolitan Cultures and Oceanic Thought*, published by Routledge (2023). His latest published work is "I Can't Breathe," a narrative artwork published in *Indian Electronic Literature Anthology* by IIT, KSHIP.

Simi Malhotra is Professor, Department of English, Jamia Millia Islamia, Delhi. Her areas of interest include literary theory and culture studies. Her latest publications are the co-edited books *Affective World-Making: Routing Planetary Thought* (Routledge, 2024), *Globalization and Sense-Making Practices: Phenomenologies of the Global, Local and Glocal* (Routledge, 2023), and *Globalization and Planetary Ethics: New Terrains of Consciousness* (Routledge, 2023); the co-authored books *Ocean as Method: Thinking with the Maritime* (Routledge, 2022) and *Terrains of Consciousness: Multilogical Perspectives on Globalization* (Würzburg University Press, 2021); and the co-edited books *Food Culture Studies in India: Consumption, Representation and Mediation*, and *Inhabiting Cyberspace in India: Theory, Perspectives and Challenges* (both from Springer, 2021).

Ruchi Nagpal has earned her doctoral degree from the Department of English, Jamia Millia Islamia. She is the co-editor of *Premchand on Literature & Life* (Routledge, 2023), along with Prof. Ameena Kazi Ansari. She has also translated more than two dozen non-fiction prose pieces of Premchand in Shuby Abidi (ed.) *Premchand on Culture and Education* (Routledge, 2021). She has authored "'Popular' and 'Classic': Deconstructing the Categories" in *Indian Popular Fiction: New Genres, Novel Spaces*, Prem Kumari Srivastava and Mona Sinha (ed.), (Routledge, 2022). She has worked as a project fellow under the aegis of UGC SAP DRS, Phase III project at the Department of English, Jamia Millia Islamia.

Sananda Roy was awarded her doctoral degree by the Department of English, Jamia Millia Islamia, and her thesis focused on Rituparno Ghosh's cinematic adaptations of a few of Tagore's works and dealt with film adaptation/translation and non-binary sexuality. She has published in several peer-reviewed journals, including a chapter in *Food Culture Studies in India: Consumption, Representation and Mediation* (Springer, 2021). She has taught at several colleges in the University of Delhi as an ad hoc assistant professor and a guest lecturer.

CONTRIBUTORS

Himanshu Balhara is a Ph.D. scholar at the Department of English, University of Delhi. His doctoral dissertation envisages "colors" as structures of cultural meaning within the celluloid medium. His research interests include classical studies, cultural studies, and comparative mythology.

James S. Baumlin is Distinguished Professor at the Department of English, Missouri State University. He has published extensively on seventeenth-century English literature (Shakespeare, Donne, and Milton) and the history of rhetoric (classical, Renaissance, and modern). He has also published widely on critical theories (classical and contemporary), composition studies, and writing pedagogy. He has won two national awards and six Missouri State awards in teaching, research, and service.

Saheli Biswas is working as Assistant Professor of English at South Calcutta Girls' College, Kolkata. She is also doing her Ph.D. on Bengali Dalit Women's writing and the understanding of cultural activism at the Centre for English Studies, Jawaharlal Nehru University, New Delhi. Her research interests include South Asian feminisms, gender and sexuality studies, and Dalit studies.

Sreerupa Bhattacharya is a Ph.D. scholar at the Indian Institute of Technology, Bombay, where she is working on women's photographic practice in twentieth-century India. Her research interests include visual culture, gender studies, technology studies, and South Asian history.

Indrani Das Gupta is Assistant Professor in the Department of English, Maharaja Agrasen College, University of Delhi. She completed her doctoral research in the field of Indian science fiction from the Department of English, Jamia Millia Islamia, New Delhi. Her articles have been published in Routledge, Bloomsbury, and Macmillan. Her recent publications include a co-edited book on Gandhi (Routledge) and chapters on Bollywood dance, Rudyard Kipling, and science fiction. She was also the fiction editor of *Mithila Review: An International Journal of Science Fiction and Fantasy*.

Vasundhara Gautam is Assistant Professor at Indraprastha College for Women, University of Delhi. She has been awarded Ph.D. at the Department of English, Jamia Millia Islamia, where she was working on "Marginalization, Identity and Representation: A Study of Haryanvi Women Folk Songs." Her areas of research interest are tribal literature and folklore, women's studies, and film studies.

Steven S. George is a Ph.D. scholar at the Department of English, Jamia Millia Islamia. He was a visiting scholar at the University of Witwatersrand, South Africa (2021–2022), and a Summer Fellow at Michigan State University, USA (2022). He has published research papers in reputed international journals and books.

Armeen Kaur Ahuja teaches English literature at Delhi University. Her research areas include performance arts, visual culture, and folklore. She is a performing artist and is committed to creating a creative school of thought within academia. Her works have been published in several books and journals and have also been commissioned by art organizations.

Gaurav Kumar is Assistant Professor of English at Shaheed Bhagat Singh College, University of Delhi. His M.Phil. dissertation submitted to the Department of Comparative Literature and Translation Studies, Ambedkar University, Delhi, examines the philosophy of desire, laughter, and translation in minor literatures of India. His research interests include comparative critical and literary theory.

Soumava Maiti is Assistant Professor of English at Techno India, Salt Lake. He completed his Ph.D. on epidemic studies/medical humanities from Delhi University and M.Phil. from Visva-Bharati, Santiniketan. He has worked as Guest Lecturer at Andul College, Calcutta University, and as a UGC Project Fellow at DU.

Sayan Parial has done his M.A. in English from the University of Gour Banga, Malda. His areas of research interest are science fiction, partition studies, posthuman studies, and science and technology studies. He is a theater practitioner at the Drama Club, University of Gour Banga.

Rashmi Sharma is a Ph.D. scholar at the Department of English and Cultural Studies, Panjab University, Chandigarh. She is pursuing her Ph.D. on the Multimodality of Graphic Representations of *Mahabharata* and their multivalent iconographic dialogue. Her area of research includes digital mythology, comics and graphic novels, and other new media interfaces, especially in the context and contour of Indian mythology.

FOREWORD

Panorama of the Pandemic: A Phenomenological Inquiry is an edited volume based on presentations made at the Young Researchers Conference organized by the Department of English, Jamia Millia Islamia from 17 to 18 December 2022. I thank Professor Simi Malhotra, Head of the Department of English, for inviting me to participate in the Conference. Professor Malhotra and her team of organizers, scholars Dr. Ruchi Nagpal, Steven S George, and Dr. Sananda Roy, have built a conference and an edited volume suited to the times. For so ambitious a project to succeed, the needful resources—curricular, technological, institutional—are substantial. Hence, my appreciation extends to Jamia Millia Islamia for supporting scholarship in the humanities.

As a collaboration among students and teachers from several universities in India and the United States, *Panorama of the Pandemic: A Phenomenological Inquiry* addresses a global audience. Beyond the timeliness of this project, I'm appreciative of the sheer range of topics/approaches and of the prominent role given to young researchers. Though we have passed through the Covid storm together, the pandemic *as an intellectual task* falls to the young researchers teaching the generations of students coming after them—students who will have grown up in a post-pandemic world, knowing no other reality.

The world has lived with Covid-19 for five years now. Over these past five years, our various institutions—scientific, medical, social, political, each "a way of seeing" and "a way of knowing"—have given us different versions of the virus. At first a mysterious killer, we see it now as a range of symptoms, some mild, some death-dealing; as a set of hospital protocols drawing on technologies available to some (not all) citizens; as a site of social-political contention over healthcare access and quality of life; as a series of mandates for social distancing and quarantine; as a debate over "individual freedom" versus "government overreach"; as a biological mutation, perhaps natural, perhaps human in origin; as an evolving sequence of viral genetic code; as an ecological "companion species," likely ineradicable, that we'll learn to live with (or else die trying). There are other versions deriving from the sciences, sociology, economics, and politics. Each remains incomplete *until given its human face*. And that's the humane task of the chapters collected here.

History is fashioned out of crises. In our time, these can be social, political, economic, ecological or, most likely, a combination thereof. Continuity within a culture is mere chronology; where nothing changes, history slumbers. For the most part, our lives are governed by common sense, habit, and the folk pathways of tradition. But, over the span of a lifetime, there comes a moment when "Mere anarchy," as Yeats puts it, "is loosed upon the world" and the old ways of thinking, feeling, speaking, and interacting with others fail.[1] Frenzied confusion ensues, gripping a community: some will hesitate in their response, having lost "conviction," while others hurl headlong on, filled with "passionate intensity." "The ceremony of innocence," as Yeats puts it, will drown. Doing damage control, we'll seek to keep some continuity in life. Left to our own devices and compelled to improvise, we'll compensate as best we can, for losses personal and collective. We are a resilient species, after all.

Such is a pattern of human history, and Covid-19 has become the crucible of change for our time. With Yeats, we might be inclined to declare "All changed, changed utterly: / A terrible beauty is born" ("Easter 1916"). For there's a sense in which our "all" *has* changed. In our politics, in our personal relationships, in our aspirations for the future, the world as we have known or imagined it is now marked by a deadly viral presence. It cohabits the planet and is here to stay. Most of us are beyond obsessing over its dangers. We allow it to retreat into the background, knowing that it can rise up at any time, in any place. In this broadly existential sense, ours has become "an age of pandemic."

Again, history is more than marking events in time, as if we lived in year 5 A.C. ("After COVID"). More than an art of memory, it's an instrument of reflection and analysis, of "making sense" of the world. Within this term is contained our capacity for storytelling: more than by facts, stats, and policy statements, our knowledge of pandemic rests in the stories gathered, told, and preserved. *These* give Covid-19 its human face, and these are the stuff of chapters collected in *Panorama of the Pandemic: A Phenomenological Inquiry*.

Following several brutal years, we have at last found some respite from the Covid storm. As infections subside within our communities, the need for action gives way to reflection; we gain distance from the crisis. Our perspective broadens, sharpens. Only now are we able to step back and, as if from higher ground, survey the pandemic-riven landscape. This wider, panoramic view is precisely what the present collection offers. Through analysis of several genres—fiction, poetry, film and theater, digital art and photography, memoir and journal writing, fieldwork reporting, and ethnography—contributors tell the stories of our time. We cannot know ourselves—where we've come from, where we're going, what we're becoming—without possession of these stories.

The chapters are wide-ranging in subject and approach, including a vision of post-anthropocentric ecology; an exploration of survival in post-apocalyptic fiction; a "plague-poetics," as developed in European novel; pandemic-inspired cyber and digital art; "pandemic photographs" (imitative of "staged" family portraits) expressing domestic loss and longing; film portrayal of caste in pandemic; pandemic themes in Haryanvi folk songs sung by women; an application of "engaged pedagogy" in the post-pandemic classroom; the racist naming of Covid variants ("Indian," "Chinese," "African"); ambivalence in application of the term, "Covid-warrior"; the euphemizing of plague/epidemic in classical Greek language and literature; traditions in the graphic representation of plague; "denial of death" as a theme in world literature; pandemic and the Indian internet's "culture of memes."[2]

Returning to Yeats's poem, "Easter 1916": if a "terrible beauty" is born from our time, surely it will be glimpsed in the artistry, wisdom, and warnings described in this collection.

James S. Baumlin
Distinguished Professor of English
Missouri State University

Notes

1 I quote from William Butler Yeats's poem, "Second Coming" (1919), which focuses on his own age's moment of crisis, when "Things fall apart":

Turning and turning in the widening gyre
The falcon cannot hear the falconer;
Things fall apart; the centre cannot hold;
Mere anarchy is loosed upon the world,
The blood-dimmed tide is loosed, and everywhere
The ceremony of innocence is drowned;
The best lack all conviction, while the worst
Are full of passionate intensity.

2 Reflecting their global perspective, the discussions of authors, artists, and film directors included Ahmed Kathadra, Manash Firaq Bhattacharjee, Emily St. John Mandel, Mary Shelley, Albert Camus, Mahima Bhayana, Anita Khemka, Imran Kokiloo, Nagraj Manjule, Dileesh Pothan, Aashiq Abu, Homer, Sophocles, Thucydides, Pieter Bruegel, Edvard Munch, Leo Tolstoy, Udayan Mukherjee, Mallika Taneja, Jorge P. Hernándes, Angela Arboleda, Jaime Núñez del Arco, Amitesh Grover, Sunita Singh, and El Pueblo. Theorists include Slavoj Žižek, Michael Polanyi, Mikhail Bakhtin, John Van Maanen, Zygmunt Bauman, Charles Rosenberg, Bernard Steigler, Brian Massumi, Gilles Deleuze and Félix Guatarri, Veena Das, Kirsten Ostherr, Ariella Azoulay, Tina Campt, Rene Girard, Michel Foucault, Lynn Margulis, Arundhati Roy, and Jacques Lacan.

ACKNOWLEDGMENTS

The compilation of *Panorama of the Pandemic: A Phenomenological Inquiry* has been a collaborative effort that has spanned several months, bringing together a diverse range of perspectives and expertise. We would like to express our deepest gratitude to all those who have contributed to this book and made this journey possible. It is a journey that is close to our hearts as it is a compilation of the enduring and excruciating experience that humankind went through during the Covid-19 pandemic. This book is dedicated to those we lost.

We would like to acknowledge the Young Researchers' Conference first and foremost, which served as the foundation for this project. It was through this conference that the idea of exploring the literary and cultural responses to the pandemic took shape. We are deeply grateful to the authors whose papers form the core of this volume. Their dedication, intellectual rigor, and passion for their respective fields, have together made this book a comprehensive exploration of the panorama of the pandemic. Their thought-provoking discussions on literature, culture, and society helped provide valuable insights into the multifaceted responses to the global crisis. Through this volume, the idea of archiving voices and perspectives on this period of momentous changes has been frozen for future academic references.

We would also like to acknowledge the unwavering support of our institution and the administrative staff of Jamia Millia Islamia. Their encouragement and resources have been invaluable throughout the course of this project.

Lastly, we would like to express our appreciation to all those who have played a part in bringing this book to fruition: whether through providing advice or assistance, or simply offering words of encouragement. We are truly grateful for your support.

Thank you

Simi Malhotra, Ruchi Nagpal, Steven S George, and Sananda Roy

INTRODUCTION

Simi Malhotra, Ruchi Nagpal,
Steven S. George, and Sananda Roy

I

In an abrupt crescendo, Covid-19 pandemic's intensity permeated the very essence of existence, effecting a profound alteration in the multifaceted framework of societal, economic, and political realms. On one axis, the advent of Covid-19 forcefully arrested the global momentum, bestowing upon humanity a somber theater of isolation and subsequent languor. Simultaneously, the pandemic's relentless march ushered in rapid metamorphoses, catalyzing an accelerated digital paradigm, exacerbating the specter of worldwide food and employment insecurity, and unleashing turbulent waves of mental health afflictions. These seismic shifts collectively birthed an emergent normalcy, echoing across the vast expanse of our shared global narrative of the pandemic.

Judith Butler in her book *What World Is This?: A Pandemic Phenomenology* (2022) suggests

> that something about the pandemic makes us reconsider the world as an object of scrutiny, register the world as a cause for alarm, mark the fact that this present version of the world was not anticipated, and see the world as suddenly bearing a new kind of opacity and imposing a new set of constraints.
>
> *(p. 13)*

This epochal realignment toward an ontological perspective of the world thus emerged as a novel paradigm, forging an unprecedented unity among individuals through a potent amalgamation brought forth by a viral agent. The perception of reality during the pandemic underwent truncation, a consequence of physical and logistical constraints imposed by diverse forms of restrictions and lockdowns.

DOI: 10.4324/9781003590392-1

Let us start by reflecting on the key term, namely, the pandemic. The etymology of the word "pandemic" is rooted in the Greek word *pandēmos* (from pan "all" + dēmos "people"). The term "pandemic," thus, includes all people and is a proposition that affects all people. The universal impact brings to mind Spinoza's distinction between *affectus* and *affectio*, the force of an affecting body and the impact it leaves on the one affected. *Affectio* may be fleeting but it may also leave a residue, a lasting impression that produces particular kinds of bodily capacities (Watkins, 2010, p. 269). In the context of the pandemic, Spinoza's distinction between *affectus* and *affectio* gained heightened significance. It delineated not only the immediate force of the pandemic's impact on individuals' body but also acknowledged the potential for enduring residues, shaping lasting bodily capacities that extend beyond the transient nature of the "affect" of the virus.

This idea ties into Spinoza's broader philosophy, particularly his concept of a fundamental connection of all beings, which he discusses at length in one of the most important, and controversial, passages in his magnum opus, *Ethics*, in 2p7 doctrine (Hübner, 2015, p. 152). Spinoza in 2p7 says,

> The order and connection of ideas is the same as the order and connection of things. (2009, p. 23) He expresses that the order and connection of ideas (in the mind) mirror the order and connection of things (in the external world). Reflecting his deterministic view—where idea of an effect is intricately connected to the cause that brought it into existence—states "thus, whether we conceive nature under the attribute of extension, or under the attribute of thought, or under any other attribute, we shall find the same order, or one and the same chain of causes—that is, the same things following in either case.
>
> *(2009, p. 24)*

This concept is fundamental to Spinoza's philosophy and has implications for understanding the interconnectedness of human beings. Butler in the context of the pandemic defines "people as porous and interconnected." She further states "The dēmos is thus not the citizens of a given state but all the people despite the legal barriers that seek to separate them or their documented status" (Butler, 2022, p. 5). The relevance of Spinoza's emphasis on the interconnectedness of individuals becomes particularly salient in the context of the pandemic. The affective experiences and traversing of individual boundaries underscore the pandemic's collective impact on humanity as a whole. This interconnectedness, central to Spinoza's metaphysical framework, highlights the integral link between human beings and their thought processes.

Moreover, this concept finds further elucidation in the context of the pandemic through Deleuze and Guattari's rhizomatic structure serving as a metaphor for a non-hierarchical, non-linear, and interconnected mode of comprehending diverse phenomena across philosophy, biology, and social organization. A rhizomatic structure, as described by Deleuze and Guattari (1987, pp. 7–8), represents a non-hierarchical, decentralized network, where connections form in multiple directions rather than following a singular, linear path. Unlike traditional root systems that have a central origin and branching points, rhizomes spread horizontally and unpredictably, exemplified by plants like bulbs and tubers, and even the behavior of animals like rats. This concept emphasizes multiplicity, movement, connectivity, and even breakout at existing dimensions, rather than adding hierarchical layers, illustrating an organic, dynamic form of growth and interaction that is always evolving. Rhizomatic in nature embodies an uncontrollable and dynamic movement, much like the behavior of a virus.

Similarly, the spread of a virus too does not adhere to any traditional hierarchical structures; it can potentially form non-linear connections across populations, and, in the course, mutate and transform itself as well as its victims, in unpredictable ways. The pandemic transcended the confines of a nation-state and other normative boundaries, placing itself within the rubric of being trans-border and cross-border as a phenomenon, unfolding in non-linear and unprecedented ways.

This global upheaval compels contemplation upon at least three profound truths to begin with. First, it underscores the inevitability and inescapability of viral intrusion; irrespective of one's social, political, or economic status, encounters with the virus remain an indomitable reality. The virus operates within a rhizomatic structure, defying hierarchies that exist in the human world. Second, it unveils an intricate interconnectedness among all of humanity. The facile inclination to isolate oneself through the constructs of nation-states and other such communal identities is radically disrupted. The Covid-19 pandemic, unlike previous predicaments, destabilized localized problems, positioning itself as a global quandary—a resonance only paralleled, albeit inadequately, by the predicament of climate change. Third, it necessitates a reimagination of our lived reality. Traditionally resistant to change, the pandemic shatters this resistance, instigating a continual alteration of realities—each day, each moment—a testament to the fragility of established constructs in the face of such unprecedented disruption.

II

The individual in the pandemic, steadfast in their resistance to the tide of change, finds himself in a perplexing paradox when forced to embrace transformation brought forth by the Covid-19 pandemic. The contemplation of this phenomenon finds its roots in the realms of confinement and isolation, where the very essence of the modern self, defined by the liberties of our age, becomes a focal point of introspection. As we navigate the uncharted waters of the pandemic, the suspension of these cherished freedoms serves as an augury, unveiling two distinct phenomena that cast a philosophical light upon human society.

First, it unveils a willingness within the individual to relinquish personal rights in exchange for the sheltering embrace of the State—a modern Leviathan guarding against the unknown, in this case, the virus. Second, it unfurls a perilous arena wherein surveillance, scrutiny, and encroachment on privacy encircle the individual like never before. Vulnerable to the State's control and regulation and its attendant measures, which, despite ostensibly claiming to favor the individual, speaks of the danger rooted in the State's all-encompassing intervention not only in the public domain but, more ominously, in the most intimate recesses of personal and private life. Thomas Hobbes, in his seminal work *Leviathan* (1981), spoke about individual rights and the social contract in great detail. In the words of Hobbes,

> The only way to erect such a common power, as may be able to defend them from the invasion of foreigners, and the injuries of one another, and thereby to secure them in such sort as that by their own industry and by the fruits of the earth they may nourish themselves and live contentedly, is to confer all their power and strength upon one man, or upon one assembly of men, that may reduce all their wills, by plurality of voices, unto one will.
>
> *(p. 54)*

Within this paradigm, sovereignty, according to Hobbes, manifests itself in the image of the Leviathan—a symbolic representation of unified and absolute power vested in a political entity. Such authority, he argues, is imperative to avert anarchy and conflict inherently present in the state of nature. Hobbes advocates the supremacy of the State, positing that any deviation from such authority would plunge society into a state of anarchy. This inherent state of disorder finds a parallel in the virus, which, if left unchecked, has the potential to unleash a form of anarchy. In a parallel exploration, Carl Schmitt's articulation in *Political Theology*

(1922) resounds: "Sovereign is he who decides on the exception" (p. 112). This statement encapsulates Schmitt's conceptualization of the "state of exception," wherein the sovereign authority possesses the prerogative to suspend ordinary laws and norms in moments of extraordinary peril, such as a threat to the very existence of the State. The resonance between seventeenth-century thinker Hobbes and twentieth-century thinker Schmitt's ideas, and the State's role during the pandemic establishes a historical and philosophical continuity, emphasizing the enduring relevance of the State's sovereignty and its all-encompassing intervention in the public and private life of individuals. The incursion into individual spheres and the potential tumult wrought by an uncontrollable viral agent engenders a compelling discourse on the dichotomy between State authority and individual autonomy in situations deemed exceptional.

In the tradition of political philosophy, Hobbes and Schmitt exalt sovereignty as paramount and position authority as supreme whereas thinkers like Agamben, Foucault, and Arendt critically question these assertions. Giorgio Agamben in his book *Where Are We Now? The Epidemic as Politics* (2021) states,

> Experience has in fact shown that, once a threat to health is in place, people are willing to accept limitations on their freedom that they would never, therefore, have considered enduring—not even during the two world wars, nor under totalitarian dictatorships.
>
> *(p. 21)*

The domain of health constitutes a pervasive sphere of human existence, wherein individuals find themselves subject to a nuanced surrender of personal entitlements in deference to the imperatives of well-being. Similarly, in the context of biopolitics, Michel Foucault articulates that the State assumes a role of governance over populations, wielding strategies and technologies to optimize life in multifaceted dimensions, encompassing health, reproduction, and collective well-being. Foucault in his *Society Must Be Defended: Lectures at the College de France, 1975–76* (2003) presents a discerning analysis and unveils a paradox inherent to the relentless pursuit of life's optimization—a propensity for the emergence of its antithesis, a realm he terms as "Thanatopolitics." Thanatopolitics, or the politics of death, materializes when the State fixates on the regulation and enhancement of life, and paradoxically veers toward practices that suppress or negate life itself. Agamben (2021), in the context of the pandemic, captures the shifting contours of citizenship in the face of the evolving biosecurity paradigm.

He articulates, "Under the new biosecurity paradigm that is being implemented before our very eyes, the idea of citizenship has completely changed, and the citizen has become the passive object of medical treatment, controls, and of all kinds of suspicion" (p. 25). The pandemic, according to Agamben, unfurls a stark reality—citizens reduced to mere biological existences, echoing an unsettling resemblance to the figure of the refugee.

In this confluence, the citizen and the refugee intertwine, as both inhabit a realm where the essence of humanity is overshadowed by the machinery of control and suspicion. Thus, one detects a sense of individuals being increasingly disenfranchised in such circumstances. Such dispossession brings to the discussion Hannah Arendt, who in her seminal work *The Origins of Totalitarianism* (1951), directs our gaze toward the dehumanizing consequences of totalitarian regimes. Through the lens of the "banality of evil," Arendt contends that ordinary individuals, acting within bureaucratic structures, can perpetrate heinous acts, exposing a chilling loss of individuality and human dignity. This, in essence, underscores a broader apprehension—a societal devaluation of life in the relentless pursuit of political or other such avowed objectives. In traversing these philosophical landscapes, a compelling argument emerges against the State's intervention in individual lives during the pandemic. The interplay of Foucault's Thanatopolitics, Arendt's cautionary accounts of totalitarian dehumanization, and Agamben's stark depiction of shifting citizenship dynamics beckon a critical examination of the ethical dimensions of State actions and the individual's role within it.

III

In this critical examination of the nature of power and its associated ubiquity, the trajectory of our inquiry leads to the idea of the "panopticon," as delineated in Foucault's *Discipline and Punish* (1977). The panopticon, as a concept, resonates beyond the confines of physical incarceration and encapsulates the expansive surveillance mechanisms threading through the fabric of society. Etymologically, the term "panopticon" emerges from the fusion of "pan," denoting "all," and "optic" derived from Greek "optikon," connoting a visual or perceptual act. In essence, the panopticon represents a State-centric modality of seeing, an optical gaze that extends ubiquitously. Simultaneously, the word "Panorama" in the title of our volume stems from the amalgamation of "pan," signifying "all," and the Greek "horama," derived from "horan," meaning "to see." Contrary to the word "optic," which conveys a hierarchical and dictatorial mode of sight, "horama" pertains to what is seen as embracing a horizontal orientation, which emerges as an assemblage and is non-linear and non-hierarchical.

The term "panorama" originates from painter Robert Barker, who, in 1792, employed it to describe his panoramic depictions of Edinburgh. The six engravings presented a 360-degree view of the city, embodying the literal essence of "a complete view." As a corollary, the juxtaposition of "optic" (hierarchical sight) and "horama" (horizontal view) underscores this inevitable contrast, of understanding how these two terms shift from hierarchical surveillance to a broader, more inclusive perspective of societal observation from their etymological roots and the political philosophy within which they are adopted. The term "pan"—"all" projects a thematic resonance throughout this volume, in the form of Spinozian "interconnectedness," Butler's critical phenomenology, and the state versus individual debate. The "pan," in the sense of all the people, becomes the core theme that delineates the critical phenomenology at the heart of our volume's exploration.

This final section of the Introduction throws light into the contextualization of the pandemic as a phenomenological phenomenon, which is a modest attempt to present a panoramic picture of the world, a comprehensive tableau of the global landscape. As the phenomenological idea of the pandemic gets contextualized, this volume attempts to probe these intersubjectivities and complex textures of social life through accounts that are rooted in expressions and narratives that allow an understanding of a worldwide crisis in its multifarious cultural and literary contexts. It becomes significant to quote Lisa Guenther, whose work on prison studies is evoked by Butler, when she says, "By critical phenomenology, I mean a method that is rooted in first-person accounts of experience but also critical of classical phenomenology's claim that the first-person singular is absolutely prior to intersubjectivity and to the complex textures of social life" (Guenther, 2013, cited in Butler, 2022, p. 71). This book is an exercise of diverging from the vertical "panopticon" to a horizontal "panorama." As a lens to capture the crushing complexities of the pandemic, this volume seeks to subvert established modes of understanding the momentous event—in order to embrace the vastness of the horizontal perspective, exploring the crisis in its diverse manifestations across the cultural and literary landscape.

A critical phenomenological inquiry is fundamentally grounded in lived experience, which is most authentically conveyed through first-hand, first-person perspectives. Sara Ahmed's *Queer Phenomenology* (2006), a profound resource for queer studies, spotlights the significance of lived experience, intentional consciousness, and the immediacy of the ready-to-hand. She posits that phenomenology places "orientation" at its core, contending that consciousness is perpetually directed "towards" an object, as it underscores the lived experience of inhabiting a body, termed by Edmund Husserl as the "living body (Leib)" (p. 2). Ahmed accentuates the impact of one's background, identity, and the encompassing world on phenomenological existence, emphasizing the entanglement within a dynamic relationship with external orientations and the proximity to objects and conditions. This living body emerging from the pandemic sees a profound reorientation of the self in tune with a renewed consciousness that is intentional. Therefore, a crisis that recenters the meaning of existence can perhaps be comprehended through the phenomenological lens, which shaped the methodology of this volume and the conference that preceded it. Through simulation of reality and the breakdown of temporalities born out of the vagaries of pandemic protocols and blurring of boundaries, we emphasize on the pandemic micro-narratives. The panoramic micro-narratives offer an expansive and multi-layered understanding of the pandemic by curating an array of perspectives, that is not only transformative but also transitional. This volume attempts to inscribe the reorientation of ontological mapping by elucidating a bricolage of accounts triggered by Covid-19.

By traversing various literary and cultural domains, these transformative transitions and articulations extend beyond conventional responses, inviting readers to envision the pandemic not as a collection of diminishing statistics but as a panoramic tableau. The panoramic lens through which the volume unfolds beckons those who have grappled with the pandemic, to glean deeper meaning from that transformative historical moment. The twofold approach adopted here combines both critical phenomenological and historical perspectives that attempt to provide a holistic view of literary and cultural works that emerged during and after the pandemic.

IV

The demonstration of intersubjectivities in the collection of chapters in this volume embodies the panoramic perspective, at times genealogically looking at the representation of pandemics and epidemics in literature and other forms of creative expressions like cinema, theater, and folk culture and at times focusing on the transformative potential of such expressions as they build a relationship between the self and the society. The first section of the volume, "Pandemic Panoramas: Narratives in the Time of Contagion," looks at literary expressions from different ages as they respond to pandemic(s) and epidemic(s). The first chapter in this section by Soumava Maiti, "Epidemic, Oriental Anxiety, and Plague

Poetics in Mary Shelley's *The Last Man*," intricately aligns with the thematic conceptualization of the book. The chapter by Maiti attempts to understand how Mary Shelley's *The Last Man* (2019) portrays a fatal fictional epidemic (plague), deconstructing the idea of Western humanism, and how they test, challenge, and undermine the post-revolutionary English as well as post-Second World War French-Algerian social, moral, religious, and political beliefs and values. In a profoundly prophetic manner, Shelley's novel becomes a premonition, set in the second half of the twenty-first century, a fictional harbinger of the Covid-19 pandemic. Shelley's world, as it crumbles owing to the pandemic—draws in its ambit, Butler's idea where the world becomes one unit, interconnected, and where the pandemic reigns—unleashing carnage regardless of hierarchies and state borders. The second chapter in this section by Rashmi Kumar, "Thy Will Be Done: Examining the Metaphysics of the Graphic Renditions of Pandemics," adeptly reflects upon the creative reactions inspired by pandemics and epidemics throughout history. This scholarly work unveils a sweeping panorama of pandemics across various epochs, engaging with the innovative medium of graphic narratives. The chapter consequently engages with the historical trajectory of graphic narratives, as they vociferously responded to pandemics and ensuing catastrophes, documenting how humans deal with such crises. The chapter becomes a practical enunciation of the theoretical idea of Thanatopolitics, redefining human's continuous quest and engagement with nature/God/death. The last chapter in the section by Indrani Dasgupta, "'Performance' of Survival in the Post-apocalyptic World: Examining Art and Academia in Emily St. John Mandel's novel *Station Eleven*," extends the realm of imagination by delving into a post-pandemic setting, contemplating on survival. Set against the backdrop of a global epidemic that decimates nearly the entire population, the novel is interpreted in the context of what contributions art and academia can make to a world and a future that exists "after the world," as it ends. The initial segment serves as a conduit that guides readers toward the contemporary crisis by employing a literary lens. This trajectory is foretold in Maiti's chapter, navigated through the discourse on pandemics and plagues as expounded in Kumar's work, and culminating in Dasgupta's chapter, which exhibits a disconcertingly prescient quality as it prognosticates a post-apocalyptic milieu. This introductory section acquaints readers with the narratives surrounding plagues and pandemics, deftly ushering them into a juncture that necessitates additional reflection and articulation.

The second section of the volume, "Philosophizing the Pandemic: Affect, Critique, and Language," presents literary output as material realities of incarceration, isolation, and its language, evoking the idea of the "pandemic" and "panorama" to look at the socio-cultural dimensions of the pandemic. The first chapter in this section by Himanshu Balhara, "Last Word: The Linguistic Response to Epidemics," charts the etymological roots of plagues and pandemics and their evolution, connoting a plethora of evolving meanings. Balhara's chapter traces the occurrences of words denoting epidemic/plague in the works of Homer, Sophocles, Thucydides, and Hippocrates and tracks the post-plague developments through Perseus Digital Library. Beyond surface-level linguistic shifts, the chapter delves into the profound implications, exploring both rational and irrational dimensions in which responses to epidemics have been documented—shedding light on historical perspectives that continue to resonate in our contemporary era. The argument of Balhara's chapter finds a contemporary echo in the next chapter in the section by Sayan Parial. Grounded in theoretical exploration, Parial's chapter, "My Race Is Not My Virus": Affective Racial Algorithms during the Covid-19 Pandemic," scrutinizes the systemic dissemination of labels such as "Indian variant," "Chinese virus," or "African variant" for the Delta variant of the coronavirus in the West. This process, orchestrated through algorithmic mass media and institutional channels, becomes imbued with symbolic and semantic racial biases against Asian, African, and South Asian diasporic communities in the West. Parial's chapter not only lays bare the entrenched racial prejudices but also endeavors to unveil the shortcomings of neoliberal care within neocapitalist states during the pandemic, by unmasking the "enclosed systems," digital affordances, and algorithms of media representations, within the "control society" of the West. The imposed restrictions as levied by the State had an innate reaction that made people question the gravity of the phenomenon delving into the arena of games acted out on social media platforms; something that the next paper in the section probes into. Gaurav Kumar's chapter, "Deathly Games: Playing in the Pandemic," delves into the unsettling trends that emerged during the pandemic, examining the phenomenon of risky behaviors such as pandemic partying and the ill-famed "TikTok Coronavirus Challenge." These brazen challenges involved individuals licking public toilet seats despite evident dangers and engaging with the concept of "death anxiety." Shedding light on these dark undertakings, the chapter critically analyzes Udayan Mukherjee's "The Party," a narrative encapsulated in *Essential Items and Other Tales from a Land in Lockdown*. This literary exploration serves as a poignant parallel to real-world occurrences, inviting readers to contemplate on the intersections of the biological and social dimensions of the pandemic. While Balhara's exposition provides a diachronic narrative elucidating the metamorphosis of language in relation to the affliction, Parial's discourse offers a synchronic exposition, anchoring the conceptualization within the contemporary milieu and explicating it through the prism of the Covid-19 pandemic. This diachronic and synchronic portrayal conveys a comprehensive panorama of the linguistic reception surrounding pandemics, with Kumar's contribution serving as a pivotal linkage that situates the discourse within the specificities of its treatment and individual responses.

Individual capacity for response gets challenged in the face of a crisis that consistently delivers itself to change. The third section titled "Pandemic Transitions: From Physical to Virtual" takes us through the transitions, liminality, contradictions, and flux that the pandemic ensued. It brings to mind Maurice Merleau-Ponty's *Phenomenology of Perception* (1962), which upholds that in delineating phenomenology, one must acknowledge that in it inheres a series of contradictions that cannot be resolved plainly and talks about the "primacy of perception," as a counter to the ontological summations of the Cartesian mind-body dualism. The body is central to Merleau-Ponty's thesis on the phenomenological structure of perception that is attributed to an intersubjective, dialectical, and intentional concept of consciousness. The first chapter in this section evokes such intersubjectivities, caught in a web of contradictions. James S. Baumlin's chapter "Teaching (in) Pandemic: Lessons Lost, Lessons Learned" rests its observations on the shoulders of dialectics, between the will to knowledge and will to ignorance, and of gain and loss, and instead posits the all-knowing as "personal." He argues that when the embodiment of experience in a physical classroom is lost as the world gets caught in the throes of a pandemic, it is but a spatial loss, a loss of bodily presence, a personal loss. As to the shared experience of the classroom, Baumlin notes: "a living, dynamic, and surprising swirl," which is "forever open to questioning and infinitely answerable," gets muted and replaced by virtual meta-narratives embodying the crisis. A lamentation along similar lines is featured in the next chapter in this section by Armeen Kaur Ahuja, titled "The Cyber in the Pandemic Art," where she opines that cyberspace fails to mimic the natural sensorium of human interaction in its simulated virtuality, as she looks at Mahima Bhayana's Art exhibition titled "16,108 Conversations between Krishna, Alexa and I," among other transitional texts, which are constitutive of the pandemic's shift to digitization. Her chapter engages with the politics of spatial liminality of cyberspace and artificial intelligence, as it seeks to redefine the origin, creation, presentation, consumption, and reception of art during the pandemic. Kaur's chapter addresses the digitization of the self through these 16,108 conversations and signposts it as a quintessentially lived experience from the lockdown.

Such digitization situates itself at the intersection of phenomenology and technology, which gets further probed by Steven S George in the next chapter in this section, titled "Digital Theatre: The Personal Is Political," which explores the transition of traditional theater into digital format, owing to physical restrictions during the pandemic. By reviewing four plays, namely, Mallika Taneja's *Allegedly*, Anuja Ghoshalkar's *The Lonely Hearts Club*, Amitesh Grover's *The Last Poet*, and Sunita Singh and El Pueblo's *No Country for Women*, the chapter enunciates how these performances have taken the "digital" and "theater" to a stage where both intersect and create an identity, that is at the same time immersive, innovative, and inquisitive. The third section delves into the theme of transitions and proffers an expansive portrayal of a global paradigm shift—transcending from conventional physical classrooms to the virtual bastions of education, as elucidated by Baumlin's treatise. The advent of the pandemic precipitated the emergence of a parallel virtual domain, encapsulating art exhibitions and theatrical presentations, a phenomenon meticulously examined by Kaur and George in the second and third papers within this section. Furthermore, this transformative wave extends its influence over crafts and artistic expressions that hitherto relied on the proximity of human interaction as an imperative for comprehending and appreciating the artistic form. These creative endeavors find themselves ensnared within the purview of the pandemic-induced transitions, unveiling unprecedented metamorphoses. As the scholarly contributions delineate these pivotal shifts, one inevitably discerns them as substantive modifications that inexorably alter the trajectory of the future.

An innovative and inquisitive identity perhaps renders itself to revolt against normative structures, which effectively encapsulates the fourth and final section of this book titled "Punctuating the Pandemic: The Audio-Visual Expressions in Covid-19" by not only curating voices crucial to exposing the deep entrenchment of caste and gender inequalities in pandemic ridden society but also experimentations with form and content that point to the liminality of spaces as markers of lived experiences during the pandemic. From the pool of literary and cultural responses that the pandemic elicited, this section looks at the context of South Asia, with particular reference to India. What has been highlighted enduringly as one reads Saheli Biswas's chapter, "Burning Hope: Caste and Pandemic in Nagraj Manjule's *Vaikunth*," is a simultaneous demonstration of Dalit abjection as one posits an aesthetic of hope. The essay discusses Dalit positions as invariably invisibilized and forced to occupy liminal spaces to underscore the phenomenology of Dalit aesthetics. As Biswas notes, Dalit aesthetics purposefully divorces itself from stylistic elegance to aver its aesthetics of unease, revolt, and dissent and argues that arts and aesthetics have always been pivotal in launching emancipatory struggles to shake off the yoke of oppression. The phenomenology of liminal spaces is offered as a contradistinction to the preceding chapter, in Sreerupa Bhattacharya's chapter titled "Shared Solitude": Reframing Family Portraits in the Time of Pandemic," which remarks on "the crafting of a liminal space," and on "the juxtaposition of different temporalities and a negotiation between presence and absence." Predicated on the photo essay "Shared Solitude" by Anita Khemka and Imran Kokiloo, Bhattacharya's chapter ekes out the aporetic nature of shared solitude, as is embodied by the staging of family portraits against backdrops incongruent with the idea of family portraits, specifically during the pandemic. The chapter dwells on the disparate categories of family portraits and the Covid-19 pandemic, thereby reorienting the reception of art, which evokes linguistic registers peculiar to the global crisis. The chapter demonstrates that from solitude to solidarity, the intersubjective gestures of one to the other, built worlds of meaning for coping and healing during the pandemic. The concluding chapter in this section by Vasundhara Gautam, titled "Lived through Covid-19 Pandemic: Understanding Lived Experience through Haryanvi Folk Songs," tries to comprehend how meaning gets generated from liminal spaces that allow for reclamation of agency by women as Gautam engages with Haryanvi folk songs on Covid-19 pandemic sung by women on digital platforms (YouTube). The chapter conjugates the content creation shift to digital platforms such as YouTube and TikTok by singers and performers during the pandemic with that of the fear and apprehensions that developed as a result of the healthcare system's collapse, to comment on the potential power of the digitized space as a tool in the hands of women to navigate the unknown terrain of Covid-19. Propelled by both facts and conspiracy theories, Covid-19 emerged as a phenomenon in its own right, unveiling catastrophic dimensions while also accentuating systemic cracks and fissures globally. The pandemic bestowed a new consciousness upon the world, intertwining it in a singular thread of humanity and engendering debates around physical health and mental well-being. This volume endeavors to scrutinize the Covid-19 pandemic through the lens of phenomenology, elucidating its transformative effects on individual and state dynamics worldwide. The ensuing collection of chapters within this volume converges diverse and singular experiences, encapsulating personal, political, and social dimensions as registers of cultural humanities attesting to the pandemic's impact. Serving as both a compendium and a gateway, this volume positions itself as a conduit for innovative, creative, and critical viewpoints across literary, cultural, pandemic, and media studies, thus contributing to the broader discourse on the multifaceted dimensions of human experience during the pandemic.

Bibliography

Agamben, G. (2021) *Where Are We Now: The Epidemic as Politics*. Translated by V. Dani. London: Eris.

Ahmed, S. (2006) *Queer Phenomenology: Orientations, Objects, Others*. Durham: Duke University Press.

Arendt, H. (1951) *The Origins of Totalitarianism*. United Kingdom: Schocken Books.

Arendt, H. (1958) *The Human Condition*. Chicago: University of Chicago Press.

Arnold, D. (2020) Pandemic India: Coronavirus and the Uses of History. *The Journal of Asian Studies*, 79(3), pp. 569–577. https://doi.org/10.1017/S0021911820002272

Barker, R. (1792) *Coloured Panorama of Edinburgh*. [Watercolour]. Scotland: University of Edinburgh, Rare Books Collections: Coll-1709.

Butler, J. (2022) *What World is This?: A Pandemic Phenomenology*. New York: Columbia University Press.

Camus, A. (1948) *The Plague*. United Kingdom: Hamish Hamilton.

Capice, K.C. and Scorsese, P. (eds.) (2022) *Pandemic Performance: Resilience, Liveness and Protest in Quarantine Times*. London and New York: Taylor and Francis.

Chaturvedi, V. (ed.) (2022) *The Pandemic: Perspectives on Asia*. Ann Arbor: Association for Asian Studies.

Deleuze, G. and Guattari, F. (1987) *A Thousand Plateaus: Capitalism and Schizophrenia*. Translated by B. Massumi. Minneapolis: University of Minnesota Press.

Foucault, M. (1977) *Discipline and Punish: The Birth of the Prison*. Translated by A. Sheridan. New York: Pantheon Books.

Foucault, M. (2003). *'Society Must Be defended': Lectures at the Collège De France, 1975–76*. Translated by D. Macey. New York: Picador.

Hobbes, T. (1981) *Leviathan*. New York: Penguin Classics.

Hübner, K. (2015) Spinoza's Parallelism Doctrine and Metaphysical Sympathy. In: E. Schliesser (ed.) *Sympathy*. London: Oxford University Press, pp. 146–170.

Merleau-Ponty, M. (1962) *Phenomenology of Perception*. Translated by C. Smith. London and New York: Routledge.

Ryan, J.M. (ed.) (2023) *COVID-19: Surviving a Pandemic*. London and New York: Routledge.

Schmitt, C. (1922) *Political Theology*. Chicago: University of Chicago Press.

Shelley, M. (2019). *The Last Man*. New York: Dover Publications.

Spinoza, B.de. (2009) *The Ethics*. Translated by R.H.M. Elwes. E-book. The Project Gutenberg. Available at: https://www.gutenberg.org/files/3800/3800-h/3800-h.htm

Völkl, Y., Obermayr, J. and Hobisch, E. (eds.) (2023) *Pandemic Protagonists: Viral (Re)Actions in Pandemic and Corona Fictions*. Bielefeld: Verlag.

Watkins, M. (2010) Desiring Recognition, Accumulating Affect. In: M. Gregg and G.J. Seigworth (eds.) *The Affect Theory Reader*. Durham: Duke University Press, pp. 269–288.

PART 1

Pandemic Panoramas

Narratives in the Time of Contagion

1

EPIDEMIC, ORIENTAL ANXIETY, AND PLAGUE POETICS IN MARY SHELLEY'S *THE LAST MAN*

Soumava Maiti

1.1 Introduction

Mary Shelley's novel *The Last Man* is set in the future and foresees how an all-devouring pandemic would annihilate the whole world except one last man, who upon his final realization about the futility of human existence discards all outward variety of appearances/illusions and becomes spiritual inside. Keeping in mind the visionary/prescient stature of the novel, this study aims to problematize and negotiate the contemporaneity of the novel in the current medical humanities research, amid the global pandemic. Vast regions of the globe underwent epidemiological crises beyond imagination, and health being a global problem, this chapter examines its paramount significance in the contemporary world.

The Last Man, a preternaturally prophetic novel that is set in the last half of the twenty-first century, revolves around the bubonic plague that eradicates the entire human race with the exception of the narrator, Lionel Verney. While writing the novel, Shelley had lessons of anatomy and disease in her mind. Contemporary magazines like *The Monthly Review* and *Blackwood Magazine* criticized the novel for its focus on the human body, physiology, and disease, particularly for its exposure of the diseased human frame bare to the public eye. Regular readers were not accustomed to the medicalized diseased bodies of the patients. *The Monthly Review* (1826) referred to it as "the offspring of a diseased imagination and of a most polluted taste" (pp. 333–335) and *Blackwood's* magazine (1827) termed it as an "abortion" (pp. 413–414).

DOI: 10.4324/9781003590392-3

The Monthly Review wrote about the novel:

> The descriptions of the operations of the pestilence are particularly objectionable for their minuteness. It is not a picture that she gives us, but a lecture in anatomy, in which every part of the *human frame is laid bare to the eye*, in its most putrid state of corruption.
>
> *(McWhir, 1996, pp. 333–335)*

From the above-mentioned quotation, it is clear how the medical ideas of anatomy, physiology, human frame, vitality, putridity, pestilence, and disease were social, moral, and political taboos for both the press and the public. In the twenty-first century with great advancements in science, technology, and medicine, it is perhaps impossible to imagine the courageous experimentation that Shelley undertook to write a novel about the pestilence and the post-pestilential apocalypse. In the truest sense, *The Last Man* is a modern piece of writing and radical in tone, since it goes beyond the popular tropes of eighteenth-century and early nineteenth-century novels. It moved beyond the popular tradition of writing, a novel about virtue and vice, sentiment and sensibility, haunted houses and terror, and at the same time about family, money, and marriage. *The Last Man* is one of the first English novels to revolve solely around the idea and notion of an epidemic—a novel where the disease is the main protagonist, against which politics of imperialism, and the ambivalent colonial relationship between the East and the West are negotiated and problematized. Although various diseases like scarlet fever, typhus, syphilis, and plague are mentioned in the text, bubonic plague is the main destructive force in the novel.

Shelley's novel is deeply rooted in the earlier discourse of disease, death, plague, power, and infection since she refers to Boccaccio, Brown, and Defoe more than once—clearly indicating the influences of *The Last Man* and the goal that the text aspires to achieve. Shelley's choice of the two cities, Constantinople and Athens, is significant, for these are one of those two ancient cities deeply associated with the disease of plague. The plague, as a deadly disease, finds its mention in *The Last Man* as an "invisible monster" (Shelley, 2008), which has its origin in Constantinople, and then spreads to Greece, Europe, America, England, and the whole world. The expansion of English militarism and politics of imperialism are possible sources of the spread of the plague. Anne McWhir (1996) conveys that "plague seems to be generated through the imposition of cultural ideals, significantly at Constantinople on the boundary of Europe and Asia, where Greek idealism and English militarism join for" (pp. 333–335). The interconnected notion of Greek idealism and British militarism is at the heart of Romantic imperialist writings, especially in the works of Lord Byron. It is not just a coincidence to note that the character of Raymond is modeled on Lord Byron.

The main characters of the novel are the narrator Lionel Verney, his sister, Perdita; Adrian and Idris, children of the last king of England; Lord Raymond; and Evadne Zaimi, a Greek princess who lives in England. In the year 2073, with the King of England's renouncement to permit the creation of an English republic, the royal family withdraws to Windsor. After many emotional and political vicissitudes, Verney marries Idris, and the hero Raymond marries Perdita. Adrian truly loves Evadne from the very beginning, but she is in love with Lord Raymond. Later, Raymond gets elected as the Lord Protector of England and immediately starts several projects for the benefit of humanity. With his sudden discovery of the Greek princess Evadne's life of misery, Raymond attempts to console his old love, though hides everything from his wife Perdita. Perdita begins suspecting her husband, and the misunderstanding between the couple becomes irreparable. Resigning his post of protectorship, Raymond leaves England to join the Greek army once again. When the Greek army is about to win the battle over the Turks with only the city of Constantinople to occupy, the besieged city becomes enormously, as well as allegorically, silent. Constantinople has fallen under the curse of the deadly plague. The armies disperse under the spell of the epidemic and the all-devouring plague starts swallowing up one and all. The aspiration of imperialism meets the fatal oriental malady, which would symbolically spread back to the heart of the Western empire. It is significant to note here that Lord Byron, on whom the character of Lord Raymond is modeled, dies from the fever that he contracts after the first and second Siege of Missolonghi. The plague starts devouring the whole of Europe with the exception of the last three survivors, who decide to leave the island to wait for death in Rome in a gentler climate. The narrator, Lionel Verney, is the lone survivor to have escaped the fatal claw of death. All alone, Verney searches for a fellow human being though in vain. He goes to Rome and spends a year writing and spiritually meditating on the future. Nobody arrives, even after Verney's long wait. Finally, he climbs St. Peter's and inscribes on a stone—"the aera 2100, last year of the world" (Shelley, 2008, p. 467, sic). Then, accompanied only by his dog, he embarks upon a spiritual journey toward an unknown space beyond the disease-ridden physical world. Verney, the only survivor of the novel, writes the "history of the last man" in Rome and with this, the novel pays homage to its most important literary precursors, Gibbon's *Decline and Fall of Roman Empire*, which Shelley read in 1815. Both Gibbon and Shelley display admiration for an imperial city on the verge of their collapse although Shelley's subject is not Rome. In *The Last Man*, Shelley undertakes the visionary task of writing about the "decline and fall of the British Empire" (Bewell, 1999, p. 297). The novel reflects on the significant role the empire has played in the global spread of disease.

1.2 Contagion and the Plague Poetics

Prior to the microbiological discoveries by Luis Pasteur and Robert Koch, medical historians agreed that there were primarily two theories of disease transmission—first, the contagionist view, which believed in a particular source of infection, named *contagiumvivum*, and which imposed the law of quarantine, and, second, the anti-contagionist miasmatic view, which identified climate and air as the source of disease. Annika Mann (2018), in her book *Reading Contagion*, succinctly notes that "*The Last Man* suggests that contagion's force cannot be localized, contained, or controlled, just as writing cannot transcend its material medium of communication, a medium that habitually infects and transforms communication itself" (p. 169). Toward the end of the novel, Verney is infected by his encounter with a black man:

> I lowered my lamp and saw a negro half clad, writhing under the agony of disease, while he held me with a convulsive grasp. With mixed horror and impatience, I strove to *disengage* myself, and fell on the sufferer; he wound his naked festering arms around me, his face was close to mine, and his breath, death-laden, entered my vitals.
>
> *(Shelley, 2008, p. 245)*

This episode powerfully dramatizes the fear of contagion as a result of the European imperialistic encounter with others, for, the encounter brings with it disease, and that's why Verney struggles to "disengage" himself from the oriental embrace of disease. Theories of contagion resist the rigidity/fixity of geographical borders because of the disruptive and transformative forces of its possible agencies like media, fomites, and collective bodies. This breaking of the map of locality and consequent global circulation of diseases had had a great influence on the "trajectory of the disease and the nature of the disease itself" (Mann, 2018, pp. 150–181). Shelley shows how the nature, trajectory, and future of any pandemic disease are intrinsically connected with the trope of imperial universalism.

Anne McWhir has a contrasting view regarding the contagious nature of the plague. Debating on the contagious and miasmatic aspects of plague, McWhir in her essay "Mary Shelley's Anti-Contagionism" contends that "Mary Shelley's emphasis on the airborne transmission of plague is metaphorically as well as medically significant, especially given her *novel's emphasis on the spread of words, ideas, and narratives*" (McWhir, 2002, p. 24, emphasis mine). Although Shelley refers to many other diseases like fever, smallpox, fever, bubonic plague, and typhus in this novel, she draws on the metaphoric meaning of plague, which is, as McWhir affirms, "any system, idea, or influence, considered to be morally or intellectually dangerous ... *The Last Man* is an infected text proliferating the destruction it describes" (McWhir, 2002, p. 24). This application of the word "infection" to "text" is intriguing. It indicates the contamination and circulation of diseased texts in the age of expansion, colonialism, and globalization. The all-devouring plague in *The Last Man*, Shelley agrees, is more attributable to the season or quality of air. Anti-contagious infectious diseases are more dangerous, for, like the exploring physicians of her age, Shelley observes that its "chief force is derived from pernicious qualities in the air, and it would probably do little harm where this was naturally salubrious" (Shelley, 2008, p. 194). Shelley uses the word "effluvia" just like Daniel Defoe's usage in *Journal of the Plague Year*, to describe the polluted/infectious malodor of diseased bodies, rotted vegetation, battlefield havoc, and wasting. Regarding the debate of the contagious or miasmatic nature of the plague, Lionel Verney, the narrator's view is quite noteworthy:

> *Nations, bordering on the already infected countries*, began to enter upon serious plans for the better keeping out of the enemy. We, commercial people, were obliged to bring such schemes under consideration; and the question of contagion became a matter of earnest disquisition. [...] That the plague was not what is commonly called contagious, like scarlet fever, or extinct smallpox, was proved.
>
> *(Shelley, 2008, p. 182, emphasis mine)*

Using the names of three deadly pestilential diseases like plague, fever, and smallpox in one sentence only testifies to Shelley's paramount concern, like the exploring physicians of her age, about the dreadful epidemics and their consequences across the globe. Amid the miasma versus contagion debates around those infectious maladies in the eighteenth and nineteenth centuries, what is significant is Shelley's consistent focus on the notion of imperialism, border-crossing, commerce, and nationalism as a recurrent motif of the spread of the pandemic. For Shelley, two constant designs in this text are the contagious/miasmatic ideas of disease and the spreading characteristic of the plague epidemic as the result of colonial travel and imperialism. In this novel, Shelley aims to depict not only the *endism* of the British Empire but also to project how the disease had been an inseparable and inevitable part of the eighteenth-century and early nineteenth-century Western enterprise of Eastward travel and colonialism. Erin O'Conner's study focuses on how contagious diseases have "operated on bodies and discourse in various historical periods" (Mann, 2018, p. 7). As a result of colonialism, globalization, and the circulation of ideas, the narrative discourses like the diseases they describe spread beyond the country of their origin. Noted critic Steven Goldsmith's succinct remark that "narrative discourse moves by touch, by contagion as it were; it 'spread'" (Shelley, 2008, p. 163) attests to the worldly quality of the disease texts. The text of *The Last Man* negotiates how the global circulation of diseases, as well as the disease narratives, exercises a shaping force on the history of imperial imagination, the history of book circulation, and the history of Romantic science.

Most plague texts have their birth in factual realities, and, therefore, in order to understand the aesthetics of plague literature, one needs to examine the transformative process from factual reality to literary reality; how the author reaches the final stage of writing through observation, perception, and experience. This journey from the perception toward the representational is very significant since this journey is not one-dimensional—it is a two-way road. Unlike Defoe's *Journal of the Plague Year* and Albert Camus's *Plague*, Shelley's *The Last Man* portrays the fictitious realities from the temporal frame of the "present." Though set in a futuristic time frame, the novel addresses contemporary issues and debates of that age like vitality, physiology, imperialism, globalization, and anxiety about the imperial epidemic. *The Last Man* is remarkable in that, within its medical explorations about the plague epidemic, it engages itself with the representational mode of co-presenting the past, present, and future.

The narrative of *The Last Man* is empirical, medical, and metaphorical. It is an allegory of the disease of human civilization in the wake of geographical expansion, colonialism, massive travels, and circulations of scientific knowledge beyond its place of origin. The narrator of Camus's *Plague* (*La Peste*), Dr. Rieux, depicts the diseased city of Oran with scientific details and day-to-day minute statistics of daily fatalities just as Defoe's narrator of *The Journal of the Plague Year*, H. F., portrays the minute detail of the plague-ridden city of London. Both the narrators engage with the social realities in the form of flesh and blood with an eye to intensify the illusion of reality. Published between Defoe's *Journal* and Camus's *Plague*, *The Last Man* pushes the concept of plague and pandemic out of its locale boundary. The reason for portraying the disease of plague in terms of globally contagious connotation in *The Last Man* is that Shelley conceives the idea of this plague as more of a political metaphor, and to her, it is a product of colonialism, globalization, and capitalism.

Rene Girard and Susan Sontag, one of the first critics to promote contagion as metaphor theory, propose to separate the metaphor of contagion from the contagion of biomedical reality. Both contagion and language have similar models of operation, the term "contagion" provides, as illustrated by Annika Mann (2018) in *Reading Contagion*, an apt model for how language itself works, and how meaning is transformed by its means of communication. Plague has long been identified as a disease of contact and communication. One thing is common in all plague texts: the textuality of plague resists every possibility of logic, rationality, and centrality/fixity of meaning—it believes in dissemination and contamination since it is uncontrollable by any border, race, or nationality. Drawing on Derrida's postulations that "[m]etaphoricity is the logic of contamination and the contamination of logic" (1981, p. 149), one can assert that metaphor is based on the logic of dissemination that infects and deconstructs the stability of definition. In plague/disease narratives there is no ultimate signifier since there are constant discussions on and references to medicalized bodies, deaths, and afterlives. The most unique thing in *The Last Man* is the philosophical meditation on a worldly journey beyond the end of the world—a worldly "appropriation" of the decayed and diseased map of the world.

The epidemic of plague in *The Last Man* is used on multi-metaphoric levels, and it breaks down the logical line between the healthy and the diseased. Both on the physical and metaphorical levels, plague is often associated with colonial expansion and "militaristic dystopias" (Cooke, 2009, p. 9). The contrast between Evadne's Hellenic ideals, and her living conditions in England is striking. When Raymond meets her, she is living in one of the most penurious streets in the metropolis. "Poverty, dirt, and squalid misery characterized its appearance" (Shelley, 2008, pp. 77–78). Evadne's life in London draws attention to the "drear and heart-sickening poverty" (Shelley, 2008, p. 78) of the urban working class. Breaking the boundary between the West and the East, she emblematizes the ambivalent and in-between epidemiological/diseased space between the two. In this novel contagion is communicated to Perdita, who shares Raymond's metaphorical sickness. Having discovered her husband's affair with Evadne, Perdita perceives their marriage from now on as a "masquerade" that "keeps up a perpetual fever in her veins ... frets her immedicable wound" (Shelley, 2008, p. 104).

With a sense of guilt and remorse, Raymond abdicates his position as Lord Protector of England and embarks on his fatal conquest of Constantinople. With Raymond's campaign for Turkish conquest, Shelley critiques the notion of Western imperialism, showing how global expansion and political power battles became the chief source of contagious epidemic diseases, and therefore the fundamental basis of the destruction of the whole world-humanity. Rather than focusing on the putrefied, natural, or contagious causes of plague, Shelley focuses on the national or political root of this pestilential disease. For Shelley, the germ of any past or future epidemic remains deep in the political greed for power and supremacy.

The description of the plague in scientific detail in plague literature is very common, but the translation of plague reality into novelistic reality is not only scientific or medical but also poetic or/and metaphorical. Just as the virus or bacillus of plague mutates constantly to escape the serum that would destroy it, so does the poetics of plague literature—which constantly addresses the new challenge, and nuances of colonialism and nationalism. Patrick Reilly in *Bills of Mortality* aptly asserts that "the plague text re-presents plague facts" (2015). The plague in the novel can be read in terms of both "specific plague" and "mythic plague" (Reilly, 2015, p. 106). Considering the ever-changing reality of the plague narrative and the challenge the novel undertakes to portray an ever-present yet futuristic reality, we can posit that in *The Last Man* "the aesthetic shifts and the metaphor is constantly reshaped" (Shelley, 2008, p. 10).[1] The linguistic metaphor of infectious plague has been always there in the literary text, particularly from the age of the Renaissance. Shakespeare used the metaphor of plague as a linguistic metaphor many times in his plays.[2] In Defoe's *Journal*, plague is used mostly as a cultural and social metaphor. True to the scientific spirit of that age, Shelley used it as a complete medical metaphor. The medical aesthetics of *The Last Man* remains in its specific focus on the interrelation among the transforming ideas of empire, politics, and medicine.

1.3 Plague, Imperialism, and Oriental Anxiety

An initial concern of the Romantic age was with the epidemic rise of disease as a result of colonial contact; many of the colonists returned home as invalids. It was getting extremely difficult to keep the two worlds (the "healthy" West and the "pathogenic" colonial world) apart. As Britain seemed to be invaded by immigrants or foreigners, the middle class was getting fearful of the epidemics. The first worldwide outbreak of cholera from 1817 to 1821 increased the ever-growing fear about the impact of international imperialism on the domestic spheres. With the news of the gradual progression of the cholera epidemic of the 1820s from the East to the West, the British people became immensely anxious about the idea that a new epidemic might appear and rapidly spread along the commercial arteries of the empire. Shelley's decision to choose plague as the central motif of the novel may have been influenced, as opined by Audrey A. Fisch (1993) in "Plaguing Politics: AIDS, Deconstruction, and *The Last Man*" by the westward progression of cholera, which "reportedly began in India." Shelley's understanding of the epidemic as a result of both colonial contact with the East and the erasure of the boundary between the East and the West is symbolically portrayed by Raymond's affair with Evadne Zaimi. The character of Evadne is referred to as the "Sultana of the East," and her upbringing is linked with "Oriental magnificence." Both Evadne and the plague are described in the novel as "foreigner/foreign." Many critics respond to the instances where the disease is referred to as a female, as "Queen of the World," which suggests that Evadne embodies as well as problematizes the idea of eastern infection. The character of Evadne is termed as a "Sultana of the East" and her upbringing is linked with "Oriental magnificence." Cynical and contemptuous of Adrian's benevolent humanitarianism, she is drawn to Raymond's desire for mastery/dominance, and he strongly intends to conquer the East. The love relation between Raymond and Evadne is clearly described in terms of colonizer/colonized or master/slave binary:

> [O]verpowered by her new sensations, she did not pause to examine them or to regulate her conduct by any sentiments except the tyrannical one which suddenly usurped the *empire of her heart*.
>
> *(Shelley, 2008, p. 31, emphasis mine)*

Thwarted in her love for Raymond, she turns her thoughts to political ambitions, returns to Greece, and plots with Russia to install her husband as ruler of Wallachia (Romania) so that she can be the princess of this realm. As the plot does not succeed, her husband commits suicide, and she is torn by an enormous sense of guilt. Having betrayed her country's emancipatory struggles, she becomes a political and social pariah in her homeland, and finally, she returns to England.

The love relation between Raymond and Evadne is very symbolic from the viewpoint of the interface between the empire and the "eastern" epidemic. With their mutual drive to rid Constantinople of Islam and Turkish influence, and to claim dominion for Europe and Christianity over the East; they ultimately unleash the plague on the entire world.

It is very intriguing to note how Shelley interweaves the theme of disease and empire in the love triangle between Perdita, Raymond, and Evadne. Shelley does not blame Raymond's sexual union with Evadne for the infection of the oriental disease; rather, it is his denial or betrayal of his wife—self-rooted deceit—that draws infection to him:

> [H]is spirit was a pure fire, which fades and shrinks from every contagion of the foul atmosphere: but now the contagion had become incorporated with its essence, and the change was more painful ... the clinging weight of destiny bent him down; he was goaded, tortured, fiercely impatient of that worst of miseries, the sense of remorse.
>
> *(Shelley, 2008, p. 91)*

Long before Lord Raymond's army besieged Constantinople, the novel insists again and again that plague has been ravaging Asia with unmatched ferocity. Lord Raymond's perversion/degeneracy in the Greek War of Independence into a war of Empire is the main reason for the annihilation of Constantinople and the dispersal of the plague, which extinguishes the whole human race. In fact, the plague appears at a significant moment in this novel, just as Lord Raymond is about to enter the deserted city of Constantinople. Raymond's conquest is inseparably enframed in egocentrism, and he is over-possessed with the idea of expelling the "antique barbarism" from Europe. Perdita, his wife, first voiced the fear of an epidemiological risk as a result of the contact with the East:

> One word, in truth, had alarmed her more than battles or seizes, during which she trusted Raymond's high command would exempt him from danger. That word, as yet it was not more to her, was PLAGUE. This enemy to the human race had begun early in June to raise its serpent-head on the shores of the Nile; parts of Asia, not usually subject to this evil, were infected.
>
> *(Shelley, 2008, p. 127)*

With the movements of armies, large pools of bodies, war, and plague are united ecologically, making possible the transmission of the disease over long distances, and at last, the plague reached Athens. Hundreds of English residents returned to their own country—the free, noble people of the most divine town in Greece fell like ripe corn before the merciless sickle of the adversary. Its pleasant places were deserted; its temples and palaces were converted into tombs; its energies ... were now forced to converge to one point, guarding against the innumerous arrows of the plague.

The plague at Athens had been preceded and caused by the contagion from the East (Shelley, 2008, p. 223). Although Europeans believed that plague was only endemic to the East, Raymond's actions for war and empire transformed the ecology of the disease since the fall of Istanbul/Constantinople blurs the boundary line between the East and the West. As a consequence, it unleashed a new virulent disease that sets sail freely across the globe—first into Thrace and Macedonia, then into Thessaly and Athens, and then toward the rest of the globe.

Adrian, who in many ways represents the novel's moral heart, recognizes clearly the brutality and reality behind Raymond's "ideal of War" (Shelley, 2008, p. 116) and refuses to "sympathize in [his] dreams of massacre and glory" (Shelley, 2008, p. 117) in spite of his commitment to the Greek cause. On the battlefield, Adrian is wounded gravely in his attempt to protect a Muslim woman from being raped by two Christian soldiers. In doing so, Shelley calls into question, by highlighting such atrocities on the part of the Greeks and Europeans, the civilizing nature of Raymond's mission as well as the whole civilizing project of European colonialism. One young Turkish soldier curses the Greeks:

> Take it, Christian dogs! take the palaces, the gardens, the mosques, the abode of our fathers—take plague with them; pestilence is the enemy we fly' if she be your friend, hug her to your bosom. The curse of Allah is on Stamboul, share ye her fate.
>
> *(Shelley, 2008, p. 191)*

The fictional pandemic is significant on psychic, moral, and political levels, and this is unfolded symbolically with the deaths of Raymond and Evadne. Evadne joined the campaign disguised as a soldier. Her dying curses at the battlefield, delivered to horrified Lionel, define imbalance and inequality of power between man and woman, self and other, colonizer and the colonized, and West and East that call forth the scourge of the plague:

> The instruments of war, fire, and the plague are my servitors. I dared, I conquered them all, till now! I have sold myself to death, with the sole condition that thou should follow now—Fire and war, and plague, unite for thy destruction ...
>
> *(Shelley, 2008, p. 131)*

In *The Last Man*, Shelley problematizes as well as negotiates with the new medical knowledge of the decayed, diseased, and precarious societies in the wake of colonial diseases in England. The plague reserves the progress of the empire. Plague is no doubt a democratizing force, which levels "all distinction of rank" (Shelley, 2008, p. 212), or as Ryland laments before Adrian—"Death and disease level all men" (Shelley, 2008, p. 244).

1.4 Plague, Globalization, and the World

> ... the library of the world is thrown to me—and in any port, I can renew my stock.
>
> (Shelley, 2008, p. 469)

The plague seems to be extremely mysterious to social and literary critics for ages; its origin and modes of transmission are obscure. Most scholars agree on the common point of plague's superiority over a national/military culture. Critics observe, as discussed earlier, that plague can spread through contagion (infected body), miasma (polluted air), and the medium of print. Both *Frankenstein* and *The Last Man* concern themselves with intra-globe travels; while Frankenstein shows its familiarity with the circulation of texts from the Orient, *The Last Man* depicts the journey of the oriental disease worldwide. Barbara Johnson (1980) is of the opinion that:

> The Plague, which extends out over the entire world from the point of encounter between East and West, is thus in a sense that which replaces the victory of the West over the East. Its lethal universality is a nightmarish version of the desire to establish a universal discourse, to spread equality and fraternity throughout the world.
>
> *(Fisch et al., 1993, p. 264)*

Unlike other plague narratives like Boccaccio's *Decameron*, Defoe's *Journal of the Plague Year*, and Charles Brockden Brown's *Arthur Mervyn* (1799), which consider disease in local terms, as part of their respective urban contexts, Shelley's *The Last Man* considers the notion of disease in "world-historical phenomena" (Bewell, 1999, p. 300). A more important influence was provided by the nineteenth-century imperial contexts, most notably the link between cholera and Hastings's Grand Army in India, and the role that disease played in the failure of Napoleon's imperial ambitions. Even Raymond confesses that his conquest of Istanbul is a repetition of Napoleon's expedition to the East. When Verney surveys the battlefield near Kishan, he sees a horrible world, ridden and wrapped up with plague and consequent deaths: "From the top of the mound, I looked far round—all was silent and deserted" (Shelley, 2008, p. 230). Shortly after Raymond's death, Verney has a dream in which his friend appears as "a gigantic phantom, bearing on its brow the sign of pestilence" (Shelley, 2008, p. 246). In his seminal work *Romanticism and Colonial Disease*, Alan Bewell aptly demonstrates that:

> Read in terms of the history of plague and the major epidemiological consequences of Britain's massive military presence in India, Shelley's identification of Raymond with the pandemic displays a profound social understanding of the dynamics of colonial disease. As a narrative in the *psychopathology of empire*, *The Last Man* articulates Britain's darkest fears, that colonialism has unleashed forces that dwarf European medical, technological, and social know-how.
>
> *(Bewell, 1999, p. 301, emphasis mine)*

Shelley is well aware of the global disaster, decay, disease, and death as the obvious consequences of the rapid expansion of colonialism in the eighteenth and nineteenth centuries. She is very cynical about "civilizing" and "improving" notions of Western imperialism. The description of England as a "vast and well-manned ship, which mastered the winds and rode proudly over the waves" (Shelley, 2008, p. 5), in the opening chapter of the novel, establishes it as an empire based on maritime trade. Despite the news that the epidemic is producing "havoc and death ... on a scale of fearful magnitude," British merchants, who are "connected with these countries," continue to trade with them. The British assumed that their scientific, commercial sophistication, agricultural, and technological development would provide immunity from this worldwide epidemic. Their hope fails ultimately, and they look to the temperateness of their seasons, placing their faith in the coming winter. All hopes were shattered with the diseased progress of time, and as a consequence of continuing trade and commerce policy whole countries as well as entire continents were demolished. Throughout the novel, Shelley gives a considerable amount of focus on the interface between the European project of colonialism, trade, and anxiety about oriental infection.

With Verney being the lone survivor meditating and future planning at the end of the novel, a palpable question confronts the readers—who is Verney? Just a narrator? The protagonist of the novel? A grim chronicler of death, disease, and pestilence? A Historian? In the nineteenth chapter of the second volume, Verney writes:

> After a long interval, I am again impelled by the restless spirit within me to continue my narration ... this journal of death; this long drawn and torturous path, leading to the ocean of countless tears, awakes me again to keen grief. I had used this *history as an opiate.*
>
> *(Shelley, 2008, p. 267)*

The expression "history as an opiate" is quite noteworthy. To the narrator of the novel also, history is a medicinal drug that can heal the history of "disease, desertion, famine, despair and death" (Shelley, 2008, p. 267). He also mentions a few books that he describes to "feed his appetite craving," and these are the accounts of "Boccaccio, De Foe, and Browne"—authors who describe in detail the "voiceless solitude of once busy earth," authors who delineate minutely the "lonely state" of diseases, plague, and death (Shelley, 2008, p. 267). Verney, like the exploring medical practitioners of that age, is a world historian or a medical historian of disease and death/end of the man who records and observes minutely the predicaments of poor and the downtrodden—"The farmers and cottagers ... struck with fear of solitude, and madly desirous of medical assistance, flocked into the towns" (Shelley, 2008, p. 269), or "the corn that sprung up in plenty, lay in autumn rotting on the ground, while the melancholy wretch who had gone out to gather bread for his children lay stiff and plague-struck in the furrow" (Shelley, 2008, p. 277), or "the ward was filled with effluvia that caused my heart to heave with painful qualms. The dead were carried out and the sick brought in, with like indifference ..." (Shelley, 2008, p. 280) and thousands of heart-rending descriptions of plague like this.

Thus, it is very interesting to note how Verney the narrator – who in the first volume of the novel was so enthusiastic about friendship, love, and passion, and described in minute detail the love triangle of Raymond-Perdita-Evadne, his own love with Idris, and Raymond's vigorous passion for the oriental conquest – becomes a sad medical historian in the middle of the narration, and from the ashes of the diseases and deaths he becomes a wanderer, seer, and self-taught philosopher. He still longs to "visit the whole extent of the earth" (Shelley, 2008, p. 468). He watches how the river Tiber spreads at his feet with many a boat "tethered to the banks" (Shelley, 2008, p. 469). He wishes to float down the stream with a few books, provisions, and his dog, and pass through the blue Mediterranean, Naples, Calabria, Scylla and Cyclades, Asia Minor, Syria, and seven-mouthed Nile. He desires to anchor in:

> another and another bay, still plowing seedless ocean, leaving behind the verdant land of native Europe, adown the tawny shore of Africa, having weathered the fierce sea of the Cape, I may moor my worn skiff in a creek, shaded by spicy groves of the odorous islands of the far Indian ocean.
>
> *(Shelley, 2008, p. 469)*

At last, he chooses his boat and takes the books of Homer and Shakespeare. The choice of Homer and Shakespeare is extremely noteworthy, since they are two classic writers whose texts travel the whole world; their writings circulate beyond the country of their origin—true to the spirit of world literature. Like the texts of Homer and Shakespeare, Verney wants his story of disease, suffering, and apocalypse to traverse the whole world beyond the western center to the marginal islands of the Indian Ocean. This apparently insignificant line from the last paragraph of the novel is extremely magical—"the library of the world is thrown to me— and in any port, I can renew my stock" (Shelley, 2008, p. 469). Dissemination of worldly knowledge and wisdom oscillates between being "thrown open" of the past and being "renewed" by the future. He moves past the physical appearance of time, for "the monotonous present" seems "intolerable" to him (Shelley, 2008, p. 470). Like the greatest philosophers of the world, he now can see past, present, and future together within the heart of time—"I shall witness all the variety of appearance, that the elements can assume" (Shelley, 2008, p. 470). He reaches this wisdom and philosophy of time, disease, and death much before the end of the novel—amid the plague, war, and pandemic—with his fundamental foreseeing—"Pestilence had become a part of our future" (Shelley, 2008, p. 270).

1.5 Conclusion

The nineteenth century is highly marked by great awareness about public health, climate, sanitation, and epidemics. It is a time when people began to reflect deeply on immunization to protect themselves from the clutches of epidemics and death. But both the doctors and the public in that era are still determining the nature of epidemics. The germ theory of disease in the last half of the nineteenth century offers a scientific basis for the epidemic outbreak. Before the advent of germ theory (around the 1870s), in the age of Romanticism, there were rigorous explorations and observations from medical practitioners. Mary Shelley's *The Last Man* is a medico-Romantic text with its particular formulation about public health, sanitation problems, and pandemics across the world.

Shelley attempts to connect medical knowledge and the need for spiritual meditation beyond the compulsive physical states of existence in the wake of the pandemic outbreak. The text endeavors to build a medical aesthetic as well as medical epistemology with its specific focus on the interface between epidemic, empire, and medical exploration. Beyond the political and imperialistic explorations, in the wake of an apocalyptic pandemic, Shelley turns the readers' attention toward the inner/spiritual exploration of the self, which the narrator attains only through his journey within and without the world.

Notes

1 While analyzing the relation between aesthetics and metaphor, the phrases "the aesthetic shifts; the metaphor is reshaped" is used by Patrick Reilly, p 10.
2 *A Midsummer Night's Dream*, *Twelfth Night.*

Bibliography

Bewell, A. (1999) *Romanticism and Colonial Disease.* Baltimore: Johns Hopkins University Press.

Blanchot, M. (1995) *Writing of the Disaster.* Translated by A. Smock. Lincoln: University of Nebraska Press.

Camus, A. (2010) *The Plague.* Translated by S. Gilbert. London: Penguin Books.

Cooke, J. (2009) *Legacies of Plague in Literature, Theory, and Film.* London: Palgrave Macmillan.

Crawfurd, R. (2021) *Plague and Pestilence in Literature and Art.* Oxford: Oxford University Press.

Defoe, D. (2010) *A Journal of the Plague Year.* Oxford: Oxford University Press.

Derrida, J. (1981) *Disseminations.* Translated by B. Johnson. London: The Athlone Press Ltd.

Fisch, A., Mellor, A.K. and Schor, E.H. (eds.) (1993). *The Other Mary Shelley.* Oxford: Oxford University Press.

Gomel, E. (2016) *The Plague of Utopias: Pestilence and the Apocalyptic Body. Twentieth-Century Literature.* Durham: Duke University Press.

Mann, A. (2018) *Reading Contagion: The Hazards of Reading in the Age of Print.* Virginia: University of Virginia Press.

McWhir, A. (ed.) (1996) *The Last Man: Mary Shelley.* Calgary: Broadview Literary Text.

McWhir, A. (2002) Mary Shelley's Anti-Contagionism: 'The Last Man' as 'Fatal Narrative'. *Mosaic: An Interdisciplinary Critical Journal*, vol. 35, no. 2, pp. 23–38. Available at: www.jstor.org/stable/44029980 (Accessed: 02 June 2024).

Reilly, P. (2015) *Bills of Mortality: Disease and Destiny in Plague Literature from Early Modern to Postmodern Times*. New York: Peter Lang Inc.

Shelley, M. (2008) *The Last Man*. Oxford: Oxford University Press.

Sontag, S. (1978) *Illness as Metaphor*. New York: Farrar, Straus, and Giroux.

2

THY WILL BE DONE[*]

Examining the Metaphysics of the Graphic Renditions of Pandemics

Rashmi Sharma

Comics or graphics are the most vestigial yet potent sites to give voice, narrative, and expression to a breadth of global experiences of the pandemic, bypassing the impactful realization of traditional antecedents of art and paintings depicting the Black Plague or the Spanish flu. Subjectivity rather than uniformity and conformability has always thrived in art. Pandemics, like art, are without borders, spawning many individualistic approaches and collective reactions. Graphics storytelling often imbues the dim reality with an emotional dimension to share an informed empathy. This allows one to see not only beyond their own circumstances and sacrifices but also elicit the perception that we may be alone in life, but in death, we are all together. Even during the Covid-19 pandemic, the cultural response to the disruption and uncertainty was most poignant in the art of comics and graphics.

These comics or graphics are testimonials of the pandemic; its narrative is composed of epidemiological maps and infographics that seek to inform, provide meaning, and illustrate the narrative of human suffering and sacrifice while providing perception and reception to process, reflect on, and understand our own befuddled experiences. These images allow one to generate not only a dynamic collective knowledge about the pandemic in a web-based cultural space but also to create, contest, embrace, and at times transform one's psyche and understanding. Comics or rather art is a visual medium and cultural commodity that have always been vital and important contributors to the visual culture of contagion, the most recent being the Covid-19 pandemic. The visual and textual properties of comics portray the nuances of the illness experienced along

* Title taken from the Bible, Gospel of Matthew, Chapter 6, Verse 10.

DOI: 10.4324/9781003590392-4

with the immediacy of a visual engagement of the world in a solitary quarantine.

Beyond the immediacy of an engagement with the visual, textual, and aesthetic properties, comics also capture the key aspects of the pandemic narrative. Pandemics transform bodily and communal spaces, and Covid-19 transformed one's social interactions and personal desires and motivations. These disruptions have always occurred concomitantly across a multitude of perspectives, be it political, social, or cultural, as well as levels of seeing from personal, national, to global, and cosmic. Art fully encapsulates the full scope and impact of a pandemic on all these levels. Visual art depicts and articulates the spatial, temporal, and relational aspects of a contagion in ways that texts may not fully represent. Throughout the history of human civilization, the outbreak of a lethal infectious disease has led to the construction of an "apocalyptic narrative" in the realm of art, which inadvertently serves to shape mankind's collective understanding of a pandemic. This narrative not only traces the social devastation and ruination but the human response to it. Unlike the Covid-19 comics, which emphasize the breakdown of geographical boundaries, how the sites confluence of infection were our own homes; the social interactions, which were physically disrupted and digitally enacted; and the desperate efforts of medical science to contain the spread and find a cure, the paintings depicting the Black Plague are more grim and pessimistic. (See *Miniature*[1] from a folio of the *Antiquitates Flandriae*, depicting the citizens of Tournai, Belgium, burying those who died of plague during the Black Death by Pierart dou Tielt (c. 1340–1360 CE), made c. 1353, and the *Triumph of Death*,[2] an oil panel painting by Pieter Bruegel the Elder painted c.1562.)

In Pierart dou Tielt's artwork, the citizens of Tournai, Belgium, are burying their dead en masse. The painting depicts 15 mourners and nine coffins all crammed together. The face of each mourner is individually highlighted, their visage conveying sorrow and fear. Similarly, in the painting titled *The Triumph of Death* by Flemish Renaissance, master Pieter Bruegel the Elder depicts the deadly catastrophe of the Black Death and how it ravaged an average European town. The blackened, desolate landscape, burning of corpses in the distance along with a sea full of shipwrecks convey that everything is dead, in flesh and spirit. The painting also depicts that people of all social backgrounds, from peasants and soldiers to nobles as well as a king and a cardinal, are equivalent in death, and the plague has taken on all of them indiscriminately. Compared to the Covid-19 comics, which depict the struggles and anxieties of people trying to cope with the pandemic, the art of the Middle Ages portrays the resignation and vanquishment of people by the plague.

In our increasingly visual society, images are a vital component of the pandemic narrative and contribute significantly to the visual culture of contagion and pathogens, as well as human anatomy. In Nunzio Paci's Visionary Anatomy painting titled *Dissected Splendor*,[3] man is depicted as caught between evisceration and rebirth and how the mutation of human anatomy in death deciphers man's relationship with nature. The Covid-19 pandemic and the art dedicated to it forced us to negotiate our relationship or rather lack of it with nature, or rather God. By harnessing the visual power of images and symbols and simultaneously depicting multiple perspectives, pandemic comics, too, delineated the social, bodily, and geographical boundaries that have been impacted by the virus. By emphasizing on the physical resilience of the human anatomy to pathogens, the social grit of coping with crumbling social interactions, and befuddled emotional responses to physical distancing, isolation, and the risk of becoming infected by your loved ones, the comics reinterpreted and anthropomorphized the human spirit or soul in graphics. Renaissance art also depicted the plague within the human social spaces and hence in direct conflict with the human spirit or impulse of life. It also articulated and legitimized the fears and anxieties of man's uneasy relationship with death, especially when it is personified as a plague (see *The Plague*[4] by Arnold Böcklin, 1898). The painting depicts Arnold Böcklin's obsession and dreary manifestations of war, pestilence, and death. As a Symbolist, his personification of Death rides on a winged creature, flying through the streets of a medieval town ravaging it with mourning and despair, as seen in the trail of bodies it left behind. Death apathy is amplified by human's helplessness against it. Similarly, a webcomic depicted Death playing snooker with Covid-19 and crumbling the world as we know it.

The pandemic comics have been the forerunner in educating, edifying, and documenting the way mankind dealt with the humanitarian crisis of death by contagion. They captured the intricate stories of personal loss, the agonies of existence, and the new terms of engagement with the social in an immediate and visceral manner. The comics via subversion of narrative, irony, and gallows humor also stealthily drew attention to the inherent prejudice and cultural biases that structure the very social fabric that we built and inhabit and reflected our social mores weakened by the pandemic. Their compelling narrative drew attention to the unacknowledged truth that mankind is its own worst enemy, and all it takes is a virus to bring it out to the fore.

Pandemic comics are also fulfilling the pedagogical function of grabbing attention to health protocols and debunking false myths relatively effortlessly due to their relatable art. Comics took the baton of informing and educating about how to prevent the spread and protect oneself and others from the contagion. The engaging visual storytelling allows the reader to identify with the experience and contextualize the impact of contagion upon one's self and environment. Comics of the Covid-19 pandemic are valuable contributions to the plague narratives and to the evolving visual culture of contagion, since the art of the Middle Ages. Art helps one to collectively process and understand this definite moment in the history of human civilization. The visual documentation of the pandemic in art not only helped to demystify the invisibility of contagion, but by creating a personal narrative even if it be of loss and suffering helped to create a sense of solidarity around shared emotions and experiences resulting from the disruptions to social interactions, bodily integrity, and communal boundaries.

While the WHO traced epidemiological routes of transmission as the virus crosses global, communal, and bodily boundaries, comics functioned as infographics to relay scientific information with their trademark humorous, irreverent, and subversive intent while acknowledging the personal and professional toll of the pandemic.[5] The medium of comics not only adds levity to distressing circumstances but also encourages one to see the bright side. They make disconcerting and emotional topics more approachable and amenable to discussion while making connections of collective memory-making. Just like we glance upon the Renaissance art to understand the Black Plague, the contemporary contributions of comics to the pandemic narrative and the visual culture of contagion shall serve as an important historical visual documentation which shall inform the future generation's understanding of both the spread of pathogens and ideas, during a pandemic.

II

The father of modern philosophy, Baruch Spinoza, was a pantheist who denied the existence of miracles nor did he believe in a God of Revelation. He considered the immutable, unchanging, and perfect laws of nature as divine. No God can interfere with nature or even a plague. Spinoza discredited free will, the distinction between good and evil, heaven and hell, and the existence of a benevolent creator who shall rescue mankind from the apocalypse. As an impious atheist with serious philosophical intent, Spinoza's understanding of God or Nature (Deus sive Natura) abetted by sound historical knowledge, a degree of literary sensitivity, and his alleged pantheism are intricately entwined with Spinoza's interpretation of God–Man relationship. In Ethics, Spinoza contended that there is only one necessarily existing, active, eternal, infinite entity that inhabits all Nature, and this is worthy of being worshipped as God. And since this God pervades everything, in substance as well as meaning then all things are God, including war, pestilence, murder, and death. Everything is conceived and destroyed in this God. Like Aristotle and Descartes, Spinoza too believed that things exist in themselves and their properties may exist in anything else. Suffering is not endemic to a pandemic alone but to war and murder as well.

Just like Sri Krishna's cosmic Vishvaroopa avatar, Spinoza's God also has incompatible properties. This God is not just permeable but also flexible and is subjected to constant change, division, and mutation, just like its many modes and properties. By continually passing through different states that differ from one another internally and in actuality, Spinoza's God is not a supremely perfect being, whose benevolence and wickedness are never constant. Hence, God is himself both the perpetrator and the victim of all the crimes and miseries of man. When a plague strikes and mankind suffers, God is, in Spinoza's account, both the plague and the suffering it causes. Spinoza also asserts that God is the immanent and not the transitive cause of all things. An immanent cause is the cause whose effects belong to or are a part of itself, like the Cartesian mind, which is said to be the cause of its own ideas. This is the cause that gives birth to itself (a virus assumes a lethal constitution for a species), whereas a transitive cause, on the other hand, brings about effects that are ontologically distinct from itself (as a virus is the cause of a pandemic). It is a cause to some effect, a reaction to an action. Spinoza deciphered God via the various properties or states assumed. By adopting the inherence interpretation, Spinoza sought to explain God's causation of things as both an immanent and a transitive causation. Émile Durkheim corroborates:

> We have only one way of demonstrating that one phenomenon is the cause of another. This is to compare the cases where they are both simultaneously present or absent, so as to discover whether the variations they display in these different combinations of circumstances provide evidence that one depends upon the other. When the phenomena can be artificially produced at will by the observer, the method is that of experimentation proper. When, on the other hand, the production of facts is something beyond our power to command, and we can only bring them together as they have been spontaneously produced, the method used is one of indirect experimentation, or the comparative method.
>
> *(Durkheim & Lukes, 1982, p. 147)*

Spinoza operates from a rather outrageous position that in nature there is nothing contingent and all things have been determined from a necessity determined by the divine nature to exist and produce an effect in a certain way, no matter how damning and devastating it may be. War, Pestilence, and Murder have been made by God in the way they manifest because they could not have been made in any other way or form. These deliberations and assertions made by Spinoza reveal him to be a necessitarian, according to whom falsity and impossibility are co-extensive. The actual world with its wars and plagues is the only possible world. Events however despicable could not have gone any differently, than the way they have gone.

Necessitarianism is at the heart of Spinoza's metaphysics and influences his views on God, inherence, causation, reason, and ontological plenitude. Since God is the only possible substance, it is impossible for any other substance which is not part of God to exist. For plague to exist necessarily, it must be conceived as being born from something that exists necessarily (Nature or God). Hence, considering the plague in relation to the rest of nature is relevant for its necessitarianism, whereas considering it as relevant in the isolated way of merely being a pestilence is not. *Undiscovered Country* (2019–), by Scott Synder and Charles Soule, is a comic that deals with plague and sickness as a part of the grim reality of isolation, mass chaos, and war in the dystopia of the United States.[6] Sickness is merely the last falling piece in a long line of dominoes and brings to the fore how the United States is crumbling under its own white supremacist zeal and violent jingoism. The trauma of death from a deadly virus to an apocalyptic zombie takeover, the graphics and panels reiterate that everything is connected and is boasted and amplified by each other. What is evident is the unraveling of the once-glorious United States of America. Part of the post-apocalyptic epic canon such as *The Walking Dead* (2010–) and *Mad Max* (1979–), and the comics, delve into man's reconciliation or submission to the pestilence and how this helplessness changes the entire humanity and its relation to Nature, and understanding the necessitarianism by which it exists. The comic attempts to negotiate the dilemma that plague has a different morality depending on the way it is endured and suffered.

The comic just like Spinoza is very pessimistic about the lack of comprehension and ability to have a conclusive idea of things, especially ones that are both a part and the whole. Spinoza laments that man's natural tendencies have failed him in grasping the comprehensive cognition of Nature and oneself. Man is hence doomed to represent objects independent of their infinitely extensive network and can never escape this contingency. For Spinoza psychology triumphs over metaphysics, and man will forever sit with his back to the sun. According to Spinoza, the mind is all-powerful and comprehends all things as necessary or vital. It has greater power over the effects of these things on human comprehension but is also immune to those seeking to influence one's morality or ethics. Pandemics push mankind to the brink of virtue where often the justification of necessitarianism offers salvation. But the anguish of such a predicament is often passive and recessive in terms of survival of the flesh and retribution of the soul. Spinoza deliberated that mankind can morally improve by recognizing, accepting, and compelling these passive affects to become part of our spiritual disposition so that man can overcome his inability to conceive finite things existing necessarily and as related to everything else. A pandemic, according to Spinoza, is an opportunity by Nature or God to improve man's prospects for moral perfection. Referring to the pandemic as a suffering for Spinoza is an expressive or conceptual incompleteness entailing falsity and denial of Nature. If each and any particular feature of the universe, considered in itself, is a dependent then their totality in culmination is also contingent (Curley, 1988, p. 49). This expansion of contingency is not a reversal of necessity. Man can only fathom the finite at a particular temporal and spatial juncture. Nature is hence elusive to even malicious since it cannot be comprehended in its entirety. This may be essentialist but a fatalist assumption of necessitarianism; it is a false one according to the reading of Spinoza. At the most expansive conceptual level (eternity), it does not jeopardize contingency at narrower levels (pandemic), so the contingency at narrower levels need not jeopardize the comprehension of things conceived in the most expansive way (Death). Egon Schiele lost his wife and unborn child to Spanish Flu, before succumbing himself. His last painting depicts his struggle to comprehend such blatant destruction of his present and future.[7] The befuddlement, the agony, and the stoic resignation of one's fate is the beginning of Spinoza's necessitarianism. Unlike Schiele artists like Arnold Böcklin and Pieter Bruegel were able to overcome the contingency and glimpse and capture the necessity of the pestilence in their art.

III

The modern and postmodern ramifications of the pandemic can be deciphered in the sociology of Zygmunt Bauman within the framework of the concept of ambivalence. Ambivalence carries within itself ambiguity, multi-meanings, chaos, and indefiniteness. The concept of ambivalence contends the concept of necessitarianism by dismantling the contentment of comprehension. Bauman contends that culture is the product of man's need to suppress his awareness of death and that it is the purpose of culture as such to conceal mortality. Since death is impossible to define since it signifies man's non-existence, man cannot conceive nor perceive one's own death, let alone see the necessity of it. So death is an absolute Nothing with no meaning. Man's fear of death is rather a fear of not existing, which was felt acutely during the Covid-19 pandemic. According to Bauman, Nothing can be perceived if perception is absent. But to perceive presence in the absence of perception is contradictive but not a flawed strategy. During the pandemic, man upon the death of loved ones experiences loss and suffering, which he also associates with his own death. But how does one experience something when one has ceased to exist altogether? Man has knowledge of his own knowledge, but no experience of his self-awareness of death.

As per Bauman, the consciousness of death is elusive and man's awareness of his own mortality is an illusion; ambivalence lies in the mere nature of thought. Thought, as contended by Spinoza, cannot fathom its own non-existence, nor can it conceive time or place that does not contain it. But Death is a state of inconceivability without thought. Pandemics reinforce that death is the real and the final truth and often a willful loss of consciousness that it is a necessity too. Bauman, like Freud, then conceives death as a spectacle that can only be viewed but never experienced, since thought ceases to exist beyond that. Death is an event where one is a spectator, present in the demise of others. Pandemic reinforced this belief. Death is also thought of as a negation of life and self, but the very act of comprehending it via thought is proof of its non-existence. The pandemic augmented many deliberations on the consciousness about mortality and how life rather than death is a traumatic experience. Hence, intention betrays thought and vice-versa. To be able to think about death after death, thought must be present in death.

Bauman's phenomenological foundations enforce that death can only be conceived by looking upon the death of others and imagining oneself in the same predicament. But imagination only generates ambivalence, not experience. Bauman also asserts that thinking about death only makes us familiar with what it is not. But the pandemic has demonstrated that negation is not denial. Death can also be a state of being. Bauman's nature of thought rests on the claim that consciousness of mortality is a more traumatic experience than death, which is never felt, only witnessed.

No Ordinary Flu (2021), a 12-page comic book on pandemic flu by Public Health, Seattle, Washington, starts with an acknowledgment of the mortality of the flesh and how individual thinking ceases to exist at the moment of one's death.[8] A kid upon coming across a photograph of his deceased uncle is enquiring about him. According to Bauman, the death of bodily existence cannot end the thought of the dead because memories like thoughts are extemporal. Set during the great pandemic of the 1918 Spanish Flu, the comic negotiates the dilemma of the body and the spirit, which are irreparably torn between mortality and immortality. Both body and spirit are ambivalent in their being because there are no reasons or even lack of reasons that give meaning to their disposition. This state of limbo is exemplified during humanitarian crises such as the pandemic.

It can be contested whether Spinoza's necessitarianism and Bauman's ambivalence of existence are crucial in understanding and even sculpting the pandemic culture. But man suffers in both the nonchalance of necessitarianism and the torment of ambivalence. Plagues bring to the fore subconscious anguish and a depressing awareness of human nature's absurdity in the face of death. But both Spinoza and Bauman confirm that human salvation is to live with meaning, worth, and purpose and a stoic forgetfulness of death. They both assert that man must be socially determined and culturally trained to believe that death is not the epilogue that must end the book of human life. What should sustain and remain is the tireless striving to give life meaning and the conscious effort to suppress the awareness of the fragility of such a meaning.

Notes

1 The image can be viewed at https://www.worldhistory.org/image/12033/citizens-of-tournai-bury-their-dead/#google_vignette.
2 The painting can be viewed at https://www.museodelprado.es/en/the-collection/art-work/the-triumph-of-death/d3d82b0b-9bf2-4082-ab04-66ed53196ccc.
3 Paintings can be viewed at https://scene360.com/art/89255/nunzio-paci/.
4 The image can be viewed at https://www.researchgate.net/figure/Webcomic-describing-the-general-impacts-of-coronavirus-pandemic-Star-Tribune-SACK-April_fig1_349699704.
5 The comics can be viewed at https://scroll.in/article/969725/how-comics-creators-are-using-the-theme-of-the-pandemic-to-depict-the-new-normal-in-everyones-lives.
6 Refer to https://imagecomics.com/comics/series/undiscovered-country.
7 See Egon Schiele, *The Family*, 1918.
8 The comic can be viewed at https://kingcounty.gov/depts/health/emergency-preparedness/preparing-yourself/pandemic-flu/~/media/depts/health/emergency-preparedness/documents/pandemic/comic-book-EN.ashx.

Bibliography

Baker, G. (2022) *Questioning: A New History of Western Philosophy*. Edinburgh: Edinburgh University Press.

Böcklin, A. (1989) *The Plague* (painting). Basel: Tempera on wood, Kunstmuseum.

Cordulack, S.W. (2002) *Edvard Munch and the Physiology of Symbolism*. Madison, [N.J.]: London: Fairleigh Dickinson University Press; Associated University Presses.

Curley, E.M. (1968) *Spinoza's Metaphysics*. Cambridge: HUP.

Curley, E.M. (1988) *Behind the Geometrical Method: A Reading of Spinoza's Ethics*. Princeton, NJ: Princeton University Press.

Darbont, Frank (dir.). (2010–2022) *The Walking Dead*.

Durkheim, E. and Lukes, S. (1982) *The Rules of Sociological Method*. New York: Free Press.

Hetrick, L.J. (2020) Embracing Uncertainty through Embracing the Arts. *Visual Arts Research*, 46(2), pp. v–vi. https://doi.org/10.5406/visuartsrese.46.2.000v

Hirsch, C.D. (2020) Pandemic Daydreams: Artist's Statement. *Feminist Studies*, 46(2), p. 327. https://doi.org/10.15767/feministstudies.46.2.0327

Hookway, N. (2017) Zygmunt Bauman's Moral Saint: Reclaiming Self in the Sociology of Morality. *Acta Sociologica*, 60(4), pp. 358–367. https://doi.org/10.1177/0001699316688947

Hviid Jacobsen, M. (2016) Zygmunt Bauman – An Ambivalent Utopian. *Revue internationale de philosophie*, 277(3), pp. 347–364. https://doi.org/10.3917/rip.277.0347

Image Comics. (n.d.) *Undiscovered Country*. [online] Available at: https://imagecomics.com/comics/series/undiscovered-country (Accessed 12 Apr. 2023).

Li Vollmer, M. and French, M. (writers), Art by Lasky, D. (2021). *No Ordinary Flu*. Seattle and King County Advanced Practice Center–Public Health.

Malabou, C. (2016) Before and Above: Spinoza and Symbolic Necessity. *Critical Inquiry*, 43(1), pp. 84–109. https://doi.org/10.1086/688294

Miller, G. and Kennedy, B. (1979) *Mad Max*. Warner Bros. Entertainment Inc.

Rocca, M.D. (2018) *The Oxford Handbook of Spinoza*. New York: Oxford University Press.

Rosenberg, C.E. (1989) Disease in History: Frames and Framers. *The Milbank Quarterly*, 67, p. 1. https://doi.org/10.2307/3350182

Silver, L. and Bruegel, P. (2011) *Pieter Bruegel*. New York: Abbeville Press Publishers.

Synder, S. and Soule, C. (2019–2024) *Undiscovered Country # 1-6*. Image Comics

Tabet, S. (2015) Zygmunt Bauman, Carlo Bordoni, State of Crisis. *Lectures*. https://doi.org/10.4000/lectures.17161

3

"PERFORMANCE" OF SURVIVAL IN A POST-APOCALYPTIC WORLD

Examining Art in Emily St. Mandel's *Station Eleven*

Indrani Das Gupta

The global outbreak of the coronavirus and its threat to human existence has forced us to reconsider our normative understanding of the world. The unfortunate consequences unleashed by the Covid-19 virus across the globe direct us to now see the world in terms of a "divide between a *before* and an *after*, a line drawn through" (Mandel, 2014, p. 20; original emphasis). If lockdowns, quarantine, health, and safety measures have become a buzzword in our encounter with modernity in the wake of the pandemic, it has also made us conscious of the unprecedented socio-political, economic, medical, cultural, and environmental crisis that has become more visible because of this disaster. This catastrophe, as Kendra Claire Capece and Patrick Scorese argue, has "underscored the precarity of systems supporting the quotidian flow of societies" (2022, p. 3). The unparalleled loss of lives and economic meltdowns across the world has made us stop in our tracks to wait, as Emily St. John Mandel states in her award-winning novel, *Station Eleven* (2014), in "fathomless silence" (p. 283). Reading Mandel's novel as evocatively depicting scenarios of the outbreak of a deadly virus to scenes where mere "survival" appears "insufficient," this essay attempts to explore the value and function of literature/artistic spaces and productions per se in a post-pandemic/post-apocalyptic world. The essay critically examines how Mandel's novel captures beauty via the force of artistic productions and spaces amid ruin and devastation. The pivotal questions the essay posits are: how are art and apocalypse related to each other? In what ways does art map social change? And does the nature or signification of artistic

DOI: 10.4324/9781003590392-5

productions undergo a transformation in the wake of a cataclysmic change?

The outbreak of the Covid-19 pandemic occasioned a global systemic failure and institutional anarchy on all fronts, from the political to the economic to cultural to social and to the disruption of gender paradigms. Yet, notwithstanding the vulnerability of the body precipitated by the global health crisis and the ongoing violence perpetrated against marginalized subjectivities caused by an almost global systemic socio-political failure, this crisis also outlined newer modes of struggle and protests. As Lynn Margulis claims, pandemics, epidemics, and evolutionary disruptions have sketched newer pathways of "evolutionary variation" (1998, p. 64). Borrowing from Margulis, this essay identifies the "evolutionary variation," as an instance of redrawing the systematized institutional violence that undergirds global modern societies. Such re-significations underlined by the pandemic have in many ways forced us to enact a more nuanced understanding of the nature of human-ness. The disastrous consequences of catastrophes like the pandemic have made us, more than ever, critically aware of how the modernist discourses like the Enlightenment centering around human agency and networks of power need to be reworked, and aligned more with a multispecies relationality to mitigate the risks inaugurated due to anthropogenic tendencies.

The "end of the world" scenario that a pandemic/cataclysmic disaster outlines facilitates imagining alternative pathways to counter climate hazards and socio-political crises brought on by the "dreams of a future that is a place of ruin" (Tate, 2017, p. 2). Positioning the essay against this backdrop of "variation" and where only "silence" is what accosts us in the face of such apocalypse, Mandel's novel is read in light of what artistic texts, artifacts, and artistic spaces could offer to the world in the future "after the world," as we know it, is no longer available.

Examining Mandel's novel as a vivid post-apocalyptic representation of the deadly fictitious Georgian Flu—"a catastrophic 'flu' that exploded like a neutron bomb over the surface of the earth" (Mandel, 2014, p. 37), this essay charts an illuminating focus away from the forces of consumerism and neo-liberal, capitalistic networks to delve into an ever-evolving utopian dream of regeneration and desire. The essay describes how in this post-pandemic world mere material depictions of life or the consumption of various artifacts or their destruction do not constitute the essential truth of life and society. Instead, as this chapter deliberates upon, it directs us to explore "the creative effort and application of knowledge" that went into producing artifacts like a science fiction graphic narrative, a museum, a photograph, a newspaper, the enactment/re-enactment of a Shakespearean drama by a traveling theatrical company in a post-apocalyptic world (Arciniega, 2021, p. 296). These various assortments of items/objects and events offer more than a collage of artistic vision underscoring "sublimity in postindustrial environments." One can argue that these artistic objects/icons/spaces are framed more in the garb of "a historical palimpsest saturated with ruins [which] signify" that the "end" is merely a myth and the systematic institutional violence and ills confronting our world have continued to proliferate (Germanà and Mousautzanis, 2014).

Through the lens of artistic denominations, this essay will explore the representation of the post-apocalyptic scenario in Mandel's novel, which, I opine, would enable us to make sense of the duality of life: whether it be in terms of life's randomness or in terms of its eternal magic. This is not to say that the essay concerns itself with providing resolutions to the preceding crisis. Instead, it engages with how disparate literary and artistic endeavors allow people to come together and "hoard memories" of the now lost "shared culture" in ordinary and at times uncanny artistic spaces and expressions (Arciniega, 2021, p. 297).

The essay is broadly divided into two sections. The first section maps the bleak and tragic sequence of events that unfolded due to the onset of the pandemic in Mandel's novel. The apocalyptic rendition of the pandemic is foregrounded via the representation of deprivation, decay, and where "hell is not other people"; rather, it is the "lack" of other people (Mandel, 2014, p. 144). This first section primarily documents the sense of loss, desolation, and utter devastation that runs parallel to the catastrophic "end of the world" scenario. Additionally, this first section resembles many popular cultural representations of catastrophes. The second section intersects with this cataclysmic representation in a way that includes a negotiation with a "finality," and concurrently intersects with a gesture of rebuttal of the very notion of "ending." This oscillation of ending or the lack of it is accounted for by verbalizing different artistic endeavors, gestures, and products that metamorphose "cultural messages" of the pre-pandemic world and redraw them in a post-pandemic world. The art flourishes in a world where the conceptual notions of national territorial borders and countries do not exist, and even basic amenities like electricity and the internet have become obsolete (Krondorfer and Karen, 2013, p. 132). In a world that is no longer a familiar space, art, as this essay argues, functions as a means not only to remember the past but also to invest those shared memories in renewing the future.

3.1 The Onset of Apocalypse: A Mediation on Loss and Decay

In different pop cultural expressions where such end-of-the-world state of affairs and apocalyptic scenarios are in vogue like *The Maze Runner* (2009–2020), *Hunger Games* (2008–10), *Interstellar* (2014), *The Last Man on Earth* (1964), and the recent Netflix show *Sweet Tooth* (2022, 2023), to name a few, the stories document a world on the brink of environmental or socio-political collapse. In many of these novels, cinematic or televised adaptations, the issue of "survival" forms the core thematic concern. These dystopian renderings offer heterogeneous representations of a post-apocalyptic era, where brutality and violence emerge as the normative pattern. The fictional representations of these futuristic worlds underscored by a pandemic/catastrophe are portrayed as devoid of a moral and institutional fabric. Additionally, such representations also direct us to redraw the assemblages of human and the non-human as the only way to survive amid the planetary crisis.

It is against this backdrop of critiquing modernity that this essay positions the reading of this novel. Emily St. John Mandel's novel, *Station Eleven*, published in 2014 and the winner of the Arthur C. Clarke Award for science fiction, is a remarkable work that intersects multiple timelines, and obliquely refers to planetary entanglements that are required to grapple with crises such as the Georgian flu pandemic depicted in the novel. However, more overtly, Mandel's novel necessitates the need to outline the role of art and artistic negotiations amid environmental disasters and the decline of the socio-political, economic, technological, and moral fabric of contemporary society. Mandel's *Station Eleven* includes numerous references to an ending, a ruin, and a disruption that cross-pollinates the present and future. Simultaneously, Mandel employs the disjointed and multiple narrative techniques in the novel to document a present whose teleological pretensions no longer hold any relevance. From describing how the outbreak of the Georgian Flu led to the "perpetual hum of the city [as] fading away" (Mandel, 2014, p. 177) to how 99 percent of the world's population was wiped out and to where gradually "countries began to go dark, city by city—no news out of Moscow, then no news out of Beijing, then Sydney, London, Paris, etc" (Mandel, 2014, p. 177), this novel literally sketches the bleakness and isolation of being alone in a world where nothing ever remains the same. While loss and ruin undergird the thematic and stylistic concern in Mandel's novel, this is not merely a representation of an existential crisis. Mandel's novel dramatizes a search for meaning, renewal, and the refusal of closure. *Station Eleven* intersects with a conceptual framework of "beauty" that undercuts the decay and disruption foregrounded through the pandemic of our contemporary world. If flows and processes of globalization have turned the whole world into a village,[1] the overwhelming presence of the iteration of the "local" in the days following the outbreak of the virus in Mandel's novel reminds us that this is a complete collapse of the socio-political, digital, and cultural ecosystem of our contemporary times:

> [T]he local news became more and more local, stations dropping away one by one, until finally the last channel on air showed only a single shot in a newsroom, station employees taking turns standing before the camera and disseminating whatever information they had, and then one night Jeevan opened his eyes at two a.m. and the newsroom was empty. Everyone had left it. [...] A day later, someone finally switched off the camera in the empty newsroom, or the camera died on its own. The day after that, the Internet blinked out.
>
> *(Mandel, 2014, p. 177)*

Technology is not merely rendered dead in this post-pandemic world but it, in the decades following the outbreak of the fictional Georgian Flu, has become part of a nihilistic dream and yet, at other times, it is also conflated with newer artistic expressions. The lack of television and the internet underlined by the catastrophic reality of the Georgian flu comments on the nightmarish dismantling of human civilizational progress, and charts a world marked by "decay, disaster and ruin" (Doyle, 2015, p. 101).

To put things into perspective, post-apocalyptic imaginaries do not merely deal with the "end of the world" scenario and the thereafter. Such fictional renderings of disaster also, as Heather Hicks rightly observes, deal with the "treatment of the episteme of modernity" (2016, p. 2). The post-apocalyptic depictions oscillate between crisis and "salvage" and provide a picture of confronting "the remnants of the modern world—from the immaterial domain of words and ideas to the physical detritus of objects and machines" (Hicks, 2016, p. 3). While apocalyptic visions, as Teresa Heffernan argues, can be seen through the lens of Christianity, marked as it is moving toward a definitive ending, post-apocalyptic narratives depict a different reality. Post-apocalyptic imaginaries showcase a frightening world that intercepts a vision of an ending while repudiating meaning and value. In post-apocalyptic narratives, the fictional renderings of the aftermath of a catastrophe also imply openness and creative possibilities (Heffernan, 2008, p. 3). In Mandel's novel, the Georgian flu catastrophe functions only as the entry point to interrogate: what should be salvaged and what ways and means lead to the process of regeneration beyond the catastrophe? And how do we assess this act of regeneration? Should we read it as an act of Christian salvation or as a Western construct of restoring order post the exit of a Paradise or merely as another exercise in meaning-making tactics?

This continual movement from representations of a ruined and blasted landscape filled with "skeleton in the driver's seat of the nearest car" (Mandel, 2014, p. 144) to enactments of Shakespeare's *King Lear* and other plays intersecting with sci-fi thematic concerns like that of Star Trek's logic of survival, and to the presence of a science fiction story, the eponymous *Station Eleven* cast in the mode of a graphic narrative to a "Museum of Civilization:" Mandel's novel is examined in this essay as a kind of metafictional text that elaborates on the value of art in changed times. While this metafictional aspect of Mandel's novel articulates a critique of the apocalyptic model of history, it also critiques the "sense-making utopian historical teleology" (De Cristofaro, 2018, p. 5) of our times.

3.2 Traces of the "Life before End": Artistic Maneuvers in Mandel's *Station Eleven*

In the novel, the theatrical traveling symphony's motto "survival is not enough" and a similar tagline engraved as a tattoo on one of the central characters, Kirsten Raymonde's arm draw our attention to the dynamic configuration of values in a post-apocalyptic setting. The tattoo/tagline of "survival is insufficient" points toward a newer delineation of post-apocalyptic renderings. Mandel's novel, in its dramatization of a melee of voices: from the sentimental to the rational, depictions of realistic settings to futuristic landscapes foregrounds how art/literature in disparate ways provides social currency to lived, embodied social relations. Mandel's novel addresses how artistic spaces, voices, and performances can function as a site of activism, "struggle, movement, and livability, while also addressing (a)liveness during a time of compounding pandemics" (Kapece and Scorese, 2022, p. 4).

The novel is broadly characterized by three timelines: 1) the events developing around the Travelling company 20 years after the devastation raged by the Georgian Flu; 2) the arrival of the flu during the night when Arthur Leander, a famous old Hollywood actor, died performing *King Lear* on the stage; 3) and the events leading up to Leander's death and especially his relationship with his ex-first wife, Miranda, who is also the writer of the science fiction graphic narrative, *Station Eleven*, and which figures as the title of this novel. Arthur's death while performing on the stage constitutes the "frame narrative" that shapes the whole novel (Feldner, 2018, p. 169). The other main characters include Kirsten, who once acted as the ghost of the younger version of Lear's daughter, Cordelia, in the same performance of *King Lear*. The other two characters are Jeevan, who was formerly a paparazzi and an entertainment journalist and is now a paramedic, and Clarke, a friend of Arthur and who was a consulting psychologist before the onset of the pandemic. During the early onset of the fictitious Georgian flu, we are told, Clarke takes it upon himself to hoard artifacts from the pre-pandemic world at a self-built "Museum of Civilization" located at the now-defunct Severn Airport. The arcs of these three central characters function as the three-pointed lens that inform the thematic and structural concerns in the novel. The essay primarily concerns itself with two of these arcs: Kristen and Clarke and their relationship to art, tradition, and the post-apocalyptic environment.

Cultural expressions in *Station Eleven* appear as a kind of transaction where our "memorie[s]" are evoked, "traded, bartered, hoarded" shared, appropriated, "and curated." A cultural artifact "acts both [as] an amulet and a shield for the [motley] survivors of the Georgia flu pandemic" (Arciniega, 2021, p. 296). These cultural artifacts shore up our familiar knowledge of culture, civilization, and values of progress while also demanding us to reinvent its values to salvage "the tangled literary and historical genomes" of our modern world (Hicks, 2016, p. 4). Drawing inspiration from Lourdes, Arciniega's reading of the overwhelming presence of artifacts in Mandel's novel as "mirroring the haphazard lives led by the protagonists whose control over their destinies unravels in the wake of the pandemic," this chapter explores the numerous artifacts being kept at the museum by Clarke or as saved by Kirsten as an illustration of the "haunting encounters" of the past with the present (Arciniega, 2021, p. 296).

The fulcrum of multiple timelines that crisscross each other draws our attention to the presence and vitality of performance aesthetics. Interestingly, the novel opens at a point when a Shakespearean theatrical performance is ongoing in a pre-pandemic world. The narrative representation of Shakespearean performance continues also in a post-pandemic world where preparations are afoot to perform a Shakespeare play in a ravaged landscape. This performativity of a Shakespearean drama constitutes, I argue, the thread of continuity that links the past, present, and future. The story begins with Arthur Leander, an aging actor, dying on the stage while performing the eponymous role of Shakespeare's *King Lear*. Even as his death due to a heart attack ironically signals the onset of the deadly Georgian flu, which destroys the world and the familiar everyday habits and rituals, Leander's death directs us to see how artistic performance and all its paraphernalia intersect with reality. The framework of performance rules large in this desolated world of *Station Eleven*. While the pandemic undercuts the control that the characters have over their lives and their future with their families being irrevocably lost with death looming large on the horizon, the continuing presence of the plastic snow that keeps on falling on the stage even after Leander's death and which co-exists with snow falling in the real world blurs the distinction between the real and the fictional. It sketches "performance," which Diana Taylor insists, as "vital acts of transfer" (2003, p. 2) of meanings, values, and memories. As said before, the multiple timelines intersect in a way that articulates Arthur as the central motif, and which is deliberated upon in other narratives The frame narrative of Arthur as an actor adapting Shakespeare, the global cultural and human civilizational icon, for the pre-epidemic socio-cultural times and the echoing presence of Arthur's fictional renditions by the Shakespearean Travelling Company draws our attention to the close interplay of artistic traditions, productions, interpretations, assimilations, and retellings. Art is here represented as contingent with the historical and socio-political tendencies, and yet its continued reverberations like the falling fake snowflakes remind us of its immense value in our times. It might not be encapsulated as truth in its literal form and yet it cannot be discounted either. Also, Arthur, Shakespeare, *King Lear*, and, subsequently, Kirsten turn out to be those material entities who offer voice to, as James Berger described, the "chaos and insignificance" that remain "trapped" "within and outside" the "boundaries" of "before and after" (1999, p. xi). The performance of the Shakespearean drama is here less a "prophecy" and more a "history" (Berger, 1999, p. xii). The continuing resonance of Shakespeare in a changed world, literally and metaphorically traveling to distant parts of the world, destabilizes the stasis that has crept in, in this "end of the world" scenario.

Chris Salter writes that the pandemic has generated a "sharpened sense of opposition between the orders of [real and fictional] experiences while also implicating [these] realms within each other in complex and contradictory ways" (cited in Walsh, 2021, p. 7). From the very beginning of the novel, Mandel represents how the act of living itself is a performance, and where artistic performance does not merely display the material world but also constitutes our realities. If Diana Taylor's famous description of performance as "transmitting social knowledge, memory, and a sense of identity" (2003, p. 2) draws our attention to how every performance frames multiple understandings of our lived experiences, Mandel's novel goes one step further. Her novel maps an encounter with the devastations caused by the pandemic to critically re-engage with our social reality. Here, transmissions of meaning and value amid ruin enacted by Kirsten's theatrical group, "Travelling Symphony," not only chalk a critical assessment of the past but simultaneously renew the future by refashioning desolated landscapes with repeated performances of Shakespeare. This Travelling Symphony recalls the ancient traditions of bards, troubadours, morality, and miracle plays, which used to move from one place to another and enact dramas from the Bible to instruct the common man about truth, justice, and love. Likewise, in Mandel's novel, this theatrical company moves from place to place to perform Shakespeare and affords a secular reinterpretation of Christian values in quotidian life. This recycling of the past in times completely different from any known vestiges of the past underscores Arthur's death as a pivotal event throughout the novel. He embodies an aesthetic semantic that encodes "a broader system of cultural representations that construct social reality" (Ryan and Kellner, 1990, p. 12). One can argue that Kirsten/Cordelia embodies the metaphorical child of Arthur/King Lear, and thus is emblematic of the "ghostly" truth that haunts a meaningless world.

Twenty years after the pandemic, we encounter Kirsten, along with a motley crew running a theatrical traveling company showcasing Shakespeare and other musicals across the ravaged settlements of Toronto. She, along with the cult leader who goes by the name of Prophet but whose real name is Tyler, and who is the son of Arthur, and the corporate consultant, Clarke, Arthur's friend, draw our attention to a critical framework of art as a "*disruptive encounter*" (De Angelis et al., 2016, p. 1; emphasis in the original). By disruptive, De Angelis et al argue for a reassessment of art underlined by the pressures of history, socio-geography, economy, politics, and ecology. Clarke's "Museum of Civilization" is not merely a repository of the lost modern world. Instead, the "Museum" functions as a new modality of an artistic convention where "the past presents itself as a contingent, interstitial and intermediate space that intervenes in the present, [but that which] brings newness to it" (De Angelis et al., 2016, p. 2). The "Museum" underlies an artistic space that refuses the dehumanization process foregrounded in the novel by the depiction of the fictitious, Georgian flu, and instead verbalizes a space of interconnectedness and a place "of becoming" (De Angelis et al., 2016, p. 4). While the trope of a museum usually entails a *stasis* underscoring of values, this is not so in Mandel's novel. The Museum built on a now-defunct airport underscores mobility even if it suggests a broken, fragmentary movement.

Interestingly, Kirsten, Tyler, and Clarke, all living in different geographical spaces, carry a copy of a graphic narrative called *Dr Eleven*, whose first volume is titled *Station Eleven*. Strikingly, this first volume carries the same name as the title of Mandel's novel "creating," according to Lourdes Arciniega, "multiple layers of textual intersection[s]" (2021, p. 296). But what is more interesting is the fact that while these characters have the same version/editions of this graphic novel, they all tend to read it differently. Clarke and Kirsten share a penchant for reinventing and reformulating the values of life in a post-apocalyptic setting via the means of curating texts/objects of various kinds. Their interpretative gestures can be identified in the context of re-envisaging history and culture. If, on the one hand, for Kirsten, with her Theatrical Travelling Symphony, survival emerges as closely affiliated with a dose of art and specifically enacting Shakespeare in an ecologically changed world. For Clarke, the museum functions as the site to curate old objects as artifacts from the pre-epidemic world like credit cards, iPhones, smartphones, laptops, and so on; signifying a gesture of remembrance of things/values/relationships we have lost. These curated "artifacts" offer an exploration into "new readings" as per Arciniega, of "the use of trauma, performance, and memory in dystopian fiction" (2021, p. 296). The Museum functions as more than a storehouse of memories. It connects the past with the present. In different ways, Kirsten and Clarke's artistic endeavors offer a glimmer of redemption and pattern from the arbitrariness of life and "the loss of historicity" (Heffernan, 2008, p. 17).

On the other hand, Tyler's understanding of the said graphic narrative is linked with networks of power. His interpretation of the graphic novel is outlined by his act of abducting a young girl from the theatrical company, who he believes is ordained to be his future wife. The marriage with this girl, Tyler believes, will increase his power manifold, and he would eventually emerge as the undisputed master of a world ravaged by an epidemic. Tyler, as a self-styled messiah of a doomsday cult, reads the epidemic as a curse from God and the survivors as committed to carry on the message of the divine. His reading of the graphic narrative leads him to invest in power, represented by his cult status (he calls himself Prophet), and underlined by his actions of killing anyone who refuses to subscribe to his values.

While Tyler's aggressive paradigm meets a sorry end, this chapter reads Kirsten and Clarke's artistic maneuvers as the only way to survive in a world where our consciousness of the world has irrevocably been shaken. Carmen M. Méndez-García (2017) argues that the survival of Shakespeare and other assorted items found in abandoned baggage at an airport "emphasizes the resilience of cultural objects in a brave new world" (p. 111) and seeks to confirm the significance of art and academia in a changed world. Describing Shakespeare and the curated items of the Museum as objects, Garcia identifies the "idea of culture" as being crucial to "defining what is human" in a changed world. However, Garcia's reading of this cultural importance in Mandel's novel is outlined as a continual projection of Anglocentric liberal humanist concerns. She reads the post-apocalyptic environment as singularly committed to "survive in an unimaginable environment." And, according to her, this survival requires the said markers of civilization, which is provided by Shakespeare functioning as the universal signifier of civilization: an ethos that will and should survive. Méndez-García (2017) claims that in the post-epidemic times when humankind has been reduced to surviving on bare essentials or "primitive order," as she claims, Shakespeare functions as a "fantasy" suggestive of the "goodness and decency in human nature, and the possibility of communal creation of little cells of camaraderie, a kind of preservation of the best of culture, society, and previous models of civilization" (p. 114). In a world where the internet, technology, and pharmaceuticals have all vanished, the remnants and reminders of what humankind imagined and created are now expressed by the singular figure of Shakespeare. Garcia finds the presence of Shakespeare as not only "cliched but [also] deeply problematic" (p. 115). She claims that the recurring motif of Shakespeare in many post-apocalyptic literary expressions like David Brin's 1985 *The Postman*, BBC's *Desert Island Discs*, and Mandel's novel, all perpetuate the idea of a universal Shakespeare, undeniably tied to the notion of Anglophonic survival. Likewise, Philip Smith goes on to exclaim that by reinventing this humanist endeavor, Mandel's novel "avoids the problematic representation of Shakespeare in the colonial encounter by presenting a world conveniently free of natives—the towns where the Traveling Symphony performs are peopled by those who have lost, and must regain, Western models of civility" (p. 301). While I agree with Garcia and Smith's concern about the reiteration of Anglocentric humanist values, I believe Mandel's novel does not conform completely to this reading. From the very beginning of the novel, the deployment of cultural artifacts and symbols like Shakespeare is underpinned by a shifting configuration of values. Aesthetic symbols, motifs, and icons, in the ruined landscape of a post-pandemic world are, I opine, metaphors that are both inside and outside history, politics, and culture. It includes the reverberations of a Christian revelation found in many apocalyptic novels and, at the same time, offers a critique of the ubiquitous paradigms of modernity—progress and a human-centric ethos. Clarke's

"Museum" and Kirsten's multiple renditions of Shakespeare in the cataclysmic landscapes of Toronto underline infinite possibilities and enunciate "the faith" in a seemingly unfamiliar world (De Cristofaro, 2020, p. 9). While Shakespeare does emerge as a central motif of culture, my understanding of the iconic figure of Shakespeare in a post-epidemic world is not outlined in a starkly black-and-white framework. The essay argues that the presence of art or the re-presencing of Shakespeare in Mandel's novel is neither cast in monolithic idiom nor governed simply by Eurocentric perspectives. Instead, Shakespeare intersects and is intercepted by other cultural objects whose meanings are continually shifting. Shakespeare operates as a text whose values are appropriated or traded with other cultural forms, and even those objects are defined differently.

The pre-eminence of Shakespeare as a cultural icon is shaken by the presence of a graphic novel, the generic assumptions of a science fiction text, and the assorted items collected from abandoned luggage found at an obscure airport alongside the presence of newspapers and photographs frayed at the edges. The tagline of the theatrical traveling symphony of Kirsten is borrowed from the popular sci-fi TV series *Star Trek* (1966–). The varying ways in which the same graphic narrative is read point toward a world that is not driven by canonical and hegemonic undertakings. Instead, the very act of reading operates as a kind of performance, and which, as the figure of Arthur in the opening pages of the novel shows, is always mutating, intersecting, and collaborating with other voices and registers. Likewise, the major characters like Kirsten, Tyler, and Clarke, all linked with the central performer, Arthur, connect in varying ways in the post-pandemic world. While Tyler and Kirsten face off at the end of the novel to rescue the abducted girl belonging to her theatrical troupe, which eventually leads to the death of Tyler, Clarke becomes aware of Kirsten's performance company via a newspaper article in the aftermath of her confrontation with Tyler; Kirsten goes to the deserted airport now transformed into a museum. Lourdes rightly argues that this novel demonstrates how everyone's actions affect others where every subjectivity remains connected with another subject mirroring the post-pandemic world devoid of borders and boundaries (2021, pp. 296–297). Here, Miranda, the first wife of Arthur and the author of the said graphic novel along with other comic book renditions that intersect with other embodied constructions and fictional enactments, refuses a parochial understanding of this changed atmosphere.

Borrowing from Joanne Freed (2017), Mandel's novel evokes a world constructed along the lines of haunting encounters where, to quote Freed, "fiction" "inspire[s] new and more ethical relationships across boundaries of difference," and which is only possible when "readers" "come into contact with others through the work of the literary imagination" (p. 31). Meetings, encounters, and confrontations in Mandel's text figure as literary expressions that operate in paradoxical ways. One can argue that Jeevan stands for the episteme of the reader, who literally and metaphorically has to intervene in the processes of narrative. Like Jeevan jumping from his position as an audience onto the stage to save Arthur, Mandel's novel demands the readers to intervene and disrupt the fixed, stable ordered meanings of art, like Shakespeare. The performance of Shakespeare and a Museum built on painstaking skills of curation do not reflect the fixity of meaning and value. Museum, as an archive, as per Katherine Hayles drawing inference from Jorge Louis Borges' story "The Aleph" opines that it is at once "part of our cultural imaginary" but also linked with matters transcendental—"can we imagine an end to the library" to "can we imagine an end to the universe." Her understanding of an archive draws attention to the role of curators who exercise "an apparatus of control" (cited in Méndez-García, 2017, p. 129). While one agrees with the image of the curator as articulating a specific remembrance of the past, Clarke's Museum built on a deserted airport and operating as a site of useless trivia—electronic objects from the pre-pandemic era points toward an ambiguous delineation of culture. Here, objects like smartphones and the like refuse the resurrection of their old meanings, and can no longer be ensconced in the changed landscape of post-pandemic, consumerist, and materialist frameworks. The curated display of objects in this "Museum of Civilization" appears as a performance similar to the Traveling Symphony's rendition of Shakespeare. Even as Clarke's controlling design signals a lost world and its attendant values, reminding the audience of the fragility of human existence, the Museum also in its enunciation of pain and trauma offers a forum "where" as Fintan Walsh observes, "performers and audiences gather to disappear and reinvent, expand and extend" (2021, p. 396).

3.3 Conclusion

While survival amid the disintegration of the known and the familiar trappings of civilization functions as the backdrop to Emily St. John Mandel's novel, *Station Eleven*, this disorienting landscape is only the beginning of a world where artistic productions and spaces function as "vehicles of integration" (Malte, 2006, p. 6). Mandel's novel refuses to subscribe only to a survival logic and underlines that merely being alive is not what will enable us to cope with the collapse of all that we are familiar with. To inhabit a post-apocalyptic world, Mandel's novel states it is important to reinvent and refashion such a world by a renewed connection and interaction with art/literature, remaking of consumerist frameworks into anesthetized spaces where "our roots are found in a shared historical and geographical space—a space filled with hurt, betrayal, and losses—[and where] we begin to bond to each other" (Krondorfer and Karen, 2013, p. 138). In post-apocalyptic scenarios, art and literature function more than an escapist dream world offering a respite from the relentless loss and crisis besetting our experiential world. Instead, as Kendra Claire Kapece and Patrick Scorese state, artistic productions manifest "as stimulants for communal engagement, not cultural or aesthetic commodities" (2022, p. 4).

Shakespeare, science fiction graphic narratives, and the Museum do not function as a fixed, stable repository of meanings. Even as stable configurations are evoked, they are immediately undercut by the juxtaposition of such cultural objects with other items. It is not a universal rendition of Shakespeare that is verbalized but an intertextual configuration of values that operates in this changed order. What becomes important in this post-epidemic world is not the object itself but a deeper understanding of artifacts proliferating in our quotidian existence and how these artifacts in their very impermanence remind us that beauty is amidst us in various ways. With the pandemic destroying public libraries and the internet becoming non-functional, Shakespeare and the objects curated in the museum are enlisted to preserve order via memories. In this fragmentary world of meaning and values undergirded by personal memories, the act of living, and grappling with a changed world, necessitates a theatrical idiom. This idiom is verbalized as collaborative and registering co-creative actions that seek to recuperate the past but in newer registers. While Tyler's superstitious delusions engraved by his mother, Elizabeth, lead to his death; his philosophical maxims are often underscored as unchangeable and non-negotiable. However, Kirsten and Clarke's assertion of culture approximates the movable stage world of the Traveling Symphony. In this unknown world, Kirsten embarks on new performances even as the old is being staged. Shakespeare intersects with forgotten histories remembered in a hazy way by Kirsten. Kirsten, who operates both as an audience and as an actor, continually explores and navigates the world around her as if for the first time. Here, the past and present intercept each other as the world unmoored in the opening pages of the novel and calls attention to things being uprooted and always moving. Miranda's paperweight, cast in the mold of capturing a storm within its structure, now belongs to Kirsten and likewise verbalizes artistic negotiations that surmount its ordinariness. The reinvention of electricity at the end of the novel is not a means to go back to the past but inaugurates a discourse of forging a community that had lost contact with each other due to the lack of internet and the closing of libraries. While Miranda's comic books figure as the most significant treasure trove for Kirsten in the post-pandemic age, it is because literature allows her to connect, as Arciniega claims, "more directly with people she has known, to lived lives to which she can relate" (2021, p. 298). Shakespeare or museums are not dead objects/spaces but operate as mechanisms to make sense of an alien world that is being fueled by our memories and reworked by our embodied experiences.

Art emerges as an intermedial space where specific meanings collate and collide while others remain in the background. It is forever-in-making, like Kirsten states to Clarke "when we come back through, I'll take this one back and leave you with the other one. That way, at least one book will always be safe" (Mandel, 2014, p. 331). Art, in *Station Eleven*, is being made and remade, appearing as a negotiable terrain that outlines moral, individual, and communal choices necessary to recover from the crisis by practicing and conserving culture. In the post-pandemic world, the written word anchors and creates a community of readers and learners. Kirsten seeks out more volumes of Miranda's *Dr. Eleven* series as a reminder of the moment when she was given the graphic novel by those she regarded as parental figures even if they were parents in the illusory and temporal world of the theater. As she wanders through the deserted towns, volumes of Miranda's handmade comic books become Kirsten's strategic maneuvers to navigate the alienated post-industrial landscape. She finds solace and empathy in reading about the lives of people who, like her, are navigating through alien worlds, be they in Hollywood or in interstellar space. Art, in Mandel's novel, appears as a cultural critique of the times we live in. But more importantly, artistic practices give voice to our fears and anxieties while also illuminating our hopes in precarious times.

Note

1 Check McLuhan's understanding of the global village.

Bibliography

Arciniega, L. (2021) Archiving the Future: The Uneasy Relationship between Individual Memory and Communal Artifacts in *Station Eleven*. *Canadian Review of Comparative Literature/Revue Canadienne de Littérature Comparée*, 48(2), pp. 296–310.

Berger, J. (1999) *After the End: Representations of Post-Apocalypse.* Minnesota: University of Minnesota Press.

De Angelis, A., Chambers, I., Celeste, I., Orabona, M. and Quadraro, M. (2016) *The Postcolonial Museum.* London and New York: Routledge.

De Cristofaro, D. (2018) Critical Temporalities: Station Eleven and the Contemporary Post-Apocalyptic Novel. *Open Library of Humanities*, 4(2):37, pp. 1–26.

De Cristofaro, D. (2020) *The Contemporary Post-Apocalyptic Novel: Critical Temporalities and the End Times.* London: Bloomsbury.

Doyle, B. (2015) The Postapocalyptic Imagination. *Thesis Eleven*, 13(1), pp. 99–113.

Feldner, M. (2018) "Survival is insufficient": The Postapocalyptic Imagination of Emily St. John Mandel's *Station Eleven. Angelica: An International Journal of English Studies*, 27(1), pp. 165–179.

Freed, J.L. (2017) *Haunting Encounters: The Ethics of Reading Across Boundaries of Difference.* New York: Cornell University Press.

Germanà, M. and Mousautzanis, A. (2014) *Apocalyptic Discourse in Contemporary Culture: Post-Millennial Perspectives on the End of the World.* London and New York: Routledge.

Heffernan, T. (2008) *Post-Apocalyptic Culture: Modernism, Postmodernism, and the Twentieth-Century Novel.* Toronto: University of Toronto Press.

Hicks, H.J. (2016) *The Post-Apocalyptic Novel in the Twenty-First Century: Modernity Beyond Salvage.* New York: Palgrave Macmillan.

Interstellar. (2014) *Film.* Directed by Christopher Nolan. USA: Paramount Pictures.

Kapece, C. and Scorese, P. (2022) *Pandemic Performance Resilience, Liveness, and Protest in Quarantine Times.* London and New York: Routledge, pp. 1–17.

Krondorfer, B. and Karen, B. (2013) From Pulp to Palimpsest: Witnessing and Re-Imagining through the Arts. In: M. Goldenberg and A. Shapiro (eds.) *Different Horrors, Same Hell: Gender and the Holocaust.* Washington: Washington Press, pp. 132–162.

Mandel, S.J. (2014) *Station Eleven.* New York and London: Harper Collins.

Margulis, L. (2013) *The Symbiotic Planet: A New Look at Evolution.* Phoenix.

McLuhan, M. and Powers, B.R. (1989) *The Global Village: Transformations in World Life and Media in the 21st Century.* Oxford: Oxford University Press.

Méndez-García, C.M. (2017) Postapocalyptic Curating: Cultural Crises and the Permanence of Art in Emily St. John Mandel's *Station Eleven. Studies in the Literary Imagination*, 50(1), pp. 111–130.

Ryan, M. and Kellner, D. (1990) *Camera Politica: The Politics and Ideology of Contemporary Hollywood Film.* Indiana: Indiana University Press.

Sweet Tooth. (2022) Television series. Created by Jim Mickle. Netflix.
Sweet Tooth. (2023) Television series. Created by Jim Mickle. Netflix.
Star Trek. (1966–) Television series. Created by Gene Roddenberry. USA: Desilu Productions
Tate, A. (2017) *Apocalyptic Fiction*. New York and London: Bloomsbury Press.
Taylor, D. (2003) *The Archive and the Repertoire: Performing Cultural Memory in the Americas*. Durham: Duke University Press.
Walsh, Fintan. (2021) Grief Machines: Transhumanist Theatre, Digital Performance, Pandemic Time. *Theatre Journal*, 73(3), pp. 391–407.

PART 2

Philosophizing the Pandemic

Affect, Critique, and Language

4

LAST WORD

The Linguistic Response to Epidemics

Himanshu Balhara

Languages are constantly changing, and evolving over time. The mythical account for the existence of a multitude of languages is enclosed within the biblical story of the Tower of Babel. In this euhemeristic vein, recent studies suggest that the earliest language or a few languages gradually changed enough to be classified into the 7,000 languages that we know of today (Leben, 2018, p. 1). The number can be expanded exponentially depending on how one counts. The study of this gradual, and other times not so gradual, process of change in language is formally known as historical linguistics. The Neo-Grammarian school of thought hypothesized that language changes according to a set number of rules that can, apart from certain select cases, always be accounted for (Hock, 1986, pp. 34–51). This school of thought is fundamentally built on a couple of influential theories that served as the impetus for historical linguistics as a legitimate discipline of study. Particularly noteworthy among some of these "laws" are Grassman's Law, Verner's Law, and especially Grimm's Law. Let us consider the latter to understand how these laws operate. Jacob Grimm, as a consequence of his project of collecting a wide variety of folk tales, stumbled upon an interesting observation. Grimm noticed a peculiarity in the specific branch of Germanic languages, which comes under the larger superstrate of Indo-European Languages. The noticeable difference in the Germanic languages, as compared to their counterparts like Latin, Greek, and Sanskrit, was the regular change of specific consonants. Grimm hypothesized that in German, the consonants like /ptk/ necessarily changed to /fθx/. So *Patēr* in Latin, *Patêr* in Greek, and *Pitā* in Sanskrit changed to *Fater* in German and ultimately Father in English, also a Germanic language (Lehmann, 1992, p. 10). If we look at a chart of IPA consonant place and manner of articulation, it is evident that the sounds move downwards in

DOI: 10.4324/9781003590392-7

the chart, or backward in the mouth. The bilabial/p/moves back to labiodental /f/, the dental /t/ to interdental /θ/, and the velar /k/ to the further glottal /x/ or [h]. Along these lines, the rest of language-change laws also operate. The Neo Grammarians, however, fail to provide the complete picture, or at least as we have it now. Winfred Lehmann notes that while such laws provide some sort of regularity to the otherwise chaotic evolution of language, they fail to account for other marked varieties of language. As it happens, the phonetic shifts of consonants as explained by these laws are only one of the drivers of language change (Lehmann, 2008, pp. 32–34). Borrowings from other languages, socio-political contexts of language evolution, and *sprachbund* linguistics, among many other topics now studied under socio-linguistics are some of the fundamental ways in which languages change (Heath, 1984, pp. 367–384). Phonological change, the one we just explained, is part of a larger system in linguistics that also includes semantic drifts, or how meanings of given words change over time. The word "fool" originally meant someone who is blessed by god. Then, it came to be associated with innocence and finally stupidity. Morphological drifts, whereby prefixes or suffixes are dropped from words, or constitute words in themselves. And syntactical change, whereby the entire sequence of words changes in a language. A prominent example of this would include the change of Old English, from an SOV language to Middle, and eventually modern English, an SVO language (Rissanen, 2008, p. 345).

This essay shall address one specific aspect of language that is often largely overlooked for its capacity to act as an agent for language change. Specifically, it shall consider taboo words, forbidden words, and censored language as drivers of language change. We'll see why there arose a need for linguistic taboos, in what context this type of language emerges, and how we, collectively as a society, work around it. While many types of categories of linguistic taboos exist, we shall focus primarily on taboos that relate to death, disease, and pestilence. In what follows, the chapter posits the argument that not only does this category comprise the strongest forms of linguistic taboos, but also, and perhaps as a consequence, it emerges as the strongest driver for language change. To this end, it examines how linguistic taboos imposed upon the demography of Athens during and after the plague years of 430 BC essentially led to a prominent instance of language change (Littman, 2009, pp. 456–467).

Taboo words or taboo language arises out of the need to avoid causing harm to oneself, or to others by way of language (Burridge and Allan, 2007, p. 9). Taboos can appear in language usually when talking about, or implicating the profane, the bodily, the sexual, the pestilent, that is, death or disease. Essentially, these are the kind of heavy-handed topics that normally we would like to circumvent around in polite company. There are a number of ways through which we can work around these linguistic taboos. We generally employ varying combinations of euphemisms, connotative language, symbolic language, metonymic language, and even non-verbal, that is, sign language to get around such taboos. At this point, it would be fruitful to establish some categories. The terms "taboo," "censoring," and "censorship" are used synonymously in general. Allan and Burridge do give a helpful distinction between censoring of language as self-imposed and censorship as state-imposed (Burridge and Allan, 2007, p. 1). The essay would further refine Burridge and Allen's distinction and posit one another important distinction, which I shall term linguistic taboos, as essentially censorship of the highest order. Before one goes on and says anything about the categories, let us be mindful of the two, perhaps central tenets of linguistics, which shall inform much of what we have to say about the categories in themselves. The first is that language is contextual. Words change meaning depending on the context in which they appear. Second, that language is arbitrary, that is, the relationship between the signifier and the signified is that of an arbitrary nature.

The first category then is what one would term "institutional censorship" of language. The restrictions placed in this category are almost always very arbitrary, highly contextual, and externally enforced. By institutional, one means, the state, which can censor language discriminating on the racial, ethnic, or the grounds of gender. The state can thus censor words that directly offend various sects under its covenant. Otherwise, the state can also censor language for propagandist purposes. Notable examples here include censorship and propaganda in Germany and Britain during the First World War. This kind of censorship, as noted, is only applicable in certain socio-political contexts and is very hard to control in the private sphere, among one's family, friends, and relatives. It is highly unlikely that this kind of censorship leads to a permanent linguistic shift when observed over a longer period of time.

The second category would be the act of self-censoring. While largely still remaining abstract to a degree, the context in self-censoring largely depends on the individual's heightened or deflated moral compass. Prominent examples in this category include cursing, swearing, and otherwise derogatory language, or politically correct language. The likelihood of adhering to, or evading, these restrictions depends upon the political inclinations, psychological makeup, and other individual markers. A study, for instance, in 2015 found that Men were comparatively more likely to swear in public than Women (Guvendir, 2015, p. 139).

The third category, which one believes to be the most tenacious form of linguistic censoring, would be Language Taboos, and it is in this sense that the term "taboo" will be used hereafter. The primary reason for the same being, one, the meaning of these taboo words remains consistent through a wide variety of contexts, as we shall see. And, two, there is a great tendency to not dissociate the signifier from the signified in these words. As stated beforehand, linguistic items that relate to either death or disease, in general, constitute the highest composition in linguistic taboos.

Let us take the example of the reconstructed proto-Indo-European word for bear, *hrtkos. As it came down to the daughter languages, the word transformed to αρχτος in Greek, ursus in Latin, and rksās in Sanskrit (Mallory and Adams, 1997, p. 55). The Greek variant denotes an association of the animal with the colder climate of the Arctic. The Latin variant derives its name from the Ursine constellation that resembles a bear, and the Sanskrit equivalent reflects the destructive capabilities of the entity, culminating in the mythological term for *Rakshasas*. Multiple works, including JP Mallory's *In Search of Indo-Europeans*, situate the *urheimet*, the homeland of Indo-European peoples in the Steppes, giving the name to the Steppe Theory (Anthony et al., 1986, pp. 291–313). If this hypothesis stands, then it would make sense for the people residing there to be fearful of the often-encountered, destructive animal that we now call "bear." In many societies, it can still be observed that the tongue holds remarkable spiritual prowess to call forth upon anything that it names (Leglise and Migge, 2006, pp. 313–339). In these societies, there are powerful naming taboos implicated within the specific cultures (Feldman, 1959, p. 237). Therefore, the name for "bear" gets displaced by a compound word in Slavic languages, translating to "honey-eater." Whereas in Germanic languages the term "bear" takes its cue from the adjective "brown," translating to something like "that brown one" (Emeneau, 1948, p. 57).

It is worth reiterating that the linguistic taboos implicated specifically in the third category are prominent because the practitioners of these taboos tend to not treat their forbidden usage as contextual, or their semiotic nature as abstract. In this case, it is highly unlikely that the original word denoting the entity gets eventually dropped out of the language and is replaced by a new word. Furthermore, it is highly likely that linguistic taboos characterized by state or self-censorship in certain social contexts get flouted on purpose. For instance, a person can deliberately flout the self-censored limitation on cursing in social contexts when they want to cause harm or insult someone in any way. State censorships can also be deliberately flouted in times of agitation or protestation against institutional policies. However, it is highly unlikely that a linguistic taboo of the third category gets flouted on purpose. The reason being that while the others are situated in a socio-political context, the nature of the third category is much more psychologically rooted in nature. There is a sense of natural law applied in this category that treads beyond the socio-political man-made laws that are tangible and erode over time.

Similarly, it is very strongly frowned upon to name the various agents of death, like dangerous, wild animals, diseases and plagues, and supernatural elements that are beyond the rationality of man like god. Different societies at different periods in history have outlawed taking the name of their respective god(s). Perhaps the most prominent instance comes from Judeo-Christian societies. Since it was considered blasphemous for Jews to directly name their God, the word was subsequently tabooed. An interesting change in language occurs as an offset of this restriction. "Yahweh," the word for God in Judaism, gets represented in writing without the use of vowels, as "YHVH." One might hypothesize that the reason for such a peculiar change in Jewish society arose owing to the prominence of the written word, the scripture, and the book in Judaism. However, when pronouncing the name out loud, they address him, not as "Yahweh" but as "Ha Shem," meaning "The Name" (Burridge and Allan, 2007, p. 38). Similarly, in Christianity, it has long been considered blasphemous to take the lord's name as it is profane, and in vain. Devout Christians would still frown upon the usage of words like "Christ," "Jesus," and "Holy." It is particularly interesting to note that while one would place these linguistic taboos, conventionally in the third category, as they deal with god, the spiritual, the unknown, and the sacerdotal. However, these taboos were enforced, quite harshly in different times by the Church as an institution. We should thus consider these words as linguistic taboos that went from the category of psychological taboos to state censorships. Naturally, as the *potestas* of the Church faded over time, so did the power of these taboos. Consequently, it was much easier to recalibrate them back into active vocabulary. It would not be surprising now to find words directly denoting God for the Judeo-Christian societies to appear in a wide array of contexts, and not just when addressing God directly.

However, unlike the semiotic nomenclature associated with God and religion, the prominence of which rises and falls with the spirit of the age, the concept of death remains ever so static. Death and disease are the one de-facto aspect that cannot be understood in any rational way, despite the overwhelming advance of science. It is with this proposition that the essay asserts that the strongest linguistic taboos occur when referring to death, diseases, illness, plagues, epidemics, and pestilence. When talking about subjects such as these, one would usually retort to euphemisms, symbolism, acronyms, assuming the symptoms of a less fatal disease, and many other ways in which one can think about working around restricted language. When talking about an illness pertaining to oneself, one often tries to understate the symptoms: statements like "under the weather," and "feeling poorly," for general illness; "upset stomach" for bouts of diarrhea; "feeling cold" or "having a cold" for a wide array of virus or bacteria-induced flu. Acronyms for diseases like "UC" for Ulcerative Colitis and "AIDS" are also prominent (Burridge and Allan, 2007, p. 99 & 156). Even among different types of disease, those that originate from respiratory or mental etiology are particularly likely to be taboo. Since respiratory diseases are most commonly perceived as infectious, they are by no means the only ones. Illness of the mind, on the other hand, has a long history of social stigmatization and exclusion from society as is carefully sketched by Foucault's well-known work *Madness and Civilization*.

Thus, the linguistic restrictions that surround the naming of death and disease primarily arise out of two kinds of irrational anxieties that intersect with each other. The first being the heightened spiritual prowess associated with naming, either animate or inanimate. Therefore, taking names of dangerous animals is forbidden in many places, as seen above. And, second, out of an irrational impulse associated with death and disease, categorizing it within the realms of the unknown. Despite the limitless progress of science and the understanding of virology, and bacteriology, death still holds that mysterious maddening frenzy that drives people to irrationality. There have been attempts to rationalize this aspect of getting sick, by attempting to portray the sick as morally corrupt. This makes getting sick a consequence of one's own actions, especially for diseases associated with sex, such as syphilis and HIV. However, the widespread outbreak of some diseases as we are now all too familiar with nulls this rationalistic tendency to associate diseases with individual moral caliber.

While countless more examples can be given and thought of regarding how languages change owing to forbidden words, it would now be beneficial to undertake an actual case study. The justification for tracking language change in Ancient Greek is two-fold. The first being that we're at a certain distance from the language, chronologically, to be able to map out the trajectory of the change. Second, since much of English vocabulary is directly borrowed from Ancient Greek, especially when concerned with medical terminology, it is worth noting that the consequence of this change remains and affects us to this day.

When we, as English speakers, think of a contagion with an infectious etiology, the first word that one can think of is perhaps an epidemic. The word "epidemic" finds its origins in the literary works of Homer over 2,500 years ago. However, neither Homer nor the subsequent prominent classical authors that make use of the term *epidemios* use it with the connotation that we are familiar with today. Instead, the terms used to describe symptoms of widespread rampant disease were *nosos* and *loimos*. *Nosos*, used first by Homer, then by Aeschylus and Plato refer to diseases, either physical, in the case of Homer, or moral corruption, in the case of Plato (Lloyd, 2003, p. 88). Sophocles in his play Oedipus Tyrannus uses the term *nosos* to refer to the physical corruption that has manifested in the city of Thebes as part of the moral corruption exhibited by Oedipus. The chorus in the play remarks, "το γαρ *νοσημα* μειζον ή ψερειν" (Sophocles, Circa 429 BC, p. 193; my emphasis) "his sickness is too great for him to bear." *Loimos* had fewer occurrences but was most frontally used to Thucydides in direct reference to the disease of the body. In the *History of the Peloponnesian War*, when describing the plague, Thucydides remarks, "οὐ μέντοι τοσοῦτός γε *λοιμὸς* οὐδὲ φθορὰ οὕτως ἀνθρώπων οὐδαμοῦ ἐμνημονεύετο γενέσθαι" (my emphasis) ("no pestilence of such an extent nor any scourge so destructive of human lives is on record anywhere") (Thucydides, 2.47.3). Robin Mitchell-Boyask hypothesizes that the subsequent disappearance of the words when referring to plagues in classical literature is a product of superstition in the aftermath of the Athenian Plague of the 430s BC (Mitchell-Boyask, 2008, pp. 374–375). I would argue instead that while Boyask is close to the point, he fails to accommodate the linguistic aspect of forbidden words in accounting for superstition.

Nosos and *loimos*, or a combination thereof, were frequently used to describe the symptoms of a contagion outbreak, or of its aftermath. The word *epidemios*, however, continued to exist and gets employed in a parallel fashion to these words but in a very different context, the least of which are medical in nature. *Epidemios* comes from the synthesis of *epi* and *deimos*. *Epi*, meaning upon, and *demos*, the people. *Epidemios*, in its earlier usage by Homer, Sophocles, and Plato, usually meant something that is spread among, or over the people. However, this usage is not exactly medical in nature. It was used almost always as a socio-economical marker, to indicate the abstract ideas of fame, justice, image, rebellion, and similar mental concepts that were spread among the demographic. In Homer's *Illiad*, for instance when Nestor in Book IX chides Agamemnon for doing wrong by Achilles, eventually he is urging Achilles to reconcile with Agamemnon. He says, "ός πολεμον επαται *επιδημιον* οκρυουεντος" ("A clan-less, lawless man he is who loves strife among his own people") (Homer, 9.64; my emphasis). Here, civil war is described *πολεμον επιδημιον*. A similar case occurs in Book 1 of the Odyssey when Athena assumes the form of Mentes to console Telemachus regarding his father's safe whereabouts. She says, "δε γαρ μιν εψανι *επιδημιον* είναι σον πατερα." ("For a true man said that he, thy father, was among his people") (Homer, 1.194; my emphasis). A few centuries later, Sophocles used the term in his play Oedipus Tyrannus to refer to rumors or bad reputation spreading among the people. In the play, when Tiresias states the prophecy to Oedipus, the chorus reminds us of the infallible reputation of Oedipus among the public as the avenger of the murdered Laius. The chorus sings, "ειμι Οιδιποδα επι ταν *επιδημον* ψάτιν," ("I could bring as proof in assailing the public reputation of Oedipus") (Sophocles, Circa 429 BC, p. 494; my emphasis).

By now, we have a very good idea of the contexts in which the usage of the word *epidemios* frequented. It was only after the later fifth century that we saw the meaning of the word develop into what we know today. The first remotely medical connotative usage of the word is associated with Hippocrates in the later part of the fifth century. Hippocrates finds himself writing right after the plague years of 430 BC, which places him as a contemporary of Thucydides. In Thucydides, we find one of the most vivid descriptions of a plague in literature. In his *History of the Peloponnesian War*, the description of the plague follows right after the Pericles' funeral oration. Thucydides description of both events gives almost the work the qualities of a classical tragic play, where both the hero and the stage are the city of Athens itself. Tracing its meteoric rise leading up to the war, culminating in its apex during the Periclean oration, the description of the plague by Thucydides is marked by a steep downfall, reminiscent of the classical tragedies. Thucydides uses a variety of words to denote both the corruption of Athens as a political body and its people as an individual body. He uses both *nosos* and *loimos* at several junctures to mean a compiled sense of death, destruction, immorality, corruption, and an irrational, almost Dionysian frenzy exhibited by the people.

Hippocrates, on the other hand, in his collection of works on medical writing, known as *Epidemics*, tries to re-establish the word *epidemios* as a replacement for collective usage of *nosos* and *loimos*, upon describing a series of symptoms spreading among the people, he says, "καιγαρ άλλος το νουσημα *επιδημος* ην." ("The disease was now spreading throughout the country") (1.1.3) (qtd. in Martin and Martin-Granel, 2006; my emphasis). Here, Hippocrates takes up an already established term *epidemios*, which, as we have seen, has been used to see the spreading of ideas or similarly abstract concepts among the masses. *Epidemios*, meaning "Upon the People," which started off as a generic ideological concept, now takes the position of specifically referring to the spread of disease, a contagion among the people, most specifically, physical in nature. It replaces, for the most part, earlier terms used to describe diseases marked by *nosos* and *loimos*.

These instances indicate that the terms *nosos* and *loimos* were used by earlier classical authors to indicate not only disease but also all of its negative syntagmatic connotations, including destruction, corruption, immorality, irrationality, and inhumanity. The idea was that individual disease and grief were thought to be brought on by a person's corrupt moral nature and thereby their impiety toward the gods. In the case of widespread plagues and epidemics, however, it is the society at large that is found corrupt and is accused of being impious in its actions (Girard, 1974, p. 833). In the usage of these terms, the authors are almost berating, and sermonizing the affected victims, indicating that the plague was brought upon them by themselves. Rather than trying to understand the contagion in terms of medical rationality, authors like Homer, Sophocles, and Thucydides try to find irrational causes for it in the actions of the victims. Although one might acquit Thucydides for his very vivid, almost pathological description of the symptoms (p. 1953). Consequently, in the *Illiad*, the plague is visibly delivered upon the people by Apollo *Smintheus*, the mouse god, in the symbolic imagery of arrows raining down from the heavens. Apollo was frequently identified with the unannounced and sudden death. This was symbolized by being shot by a single arrow by Apollo. Therefore, the raining down of arrows in a flurry represents the unknown etiology of the plague in the bronze age world of Troy, gripping everyone by the masses, much akin to a sudden cardiac arrest (Bernheim and Zener, 1978, pp. 11–14). Furthermore, the anxiety associated with the oblivious origins of the plague culminates in being placed within a moral and ethical circumference. It is quite clearly stated in the epic that the plague was a direct consequence of affronting the Gods. In Book I, the Greeks in the Trojan War take captive an Apollonian Priest's daughter as *τιμη*, or spoils of war. Doing so angers Apollo, associated not only with healing and music but also with plague and disease. In Sophocles, the city of Thebes is condemned with a plague, as their leader, Oedipus, is burdened with miasmic corruption, a sin, albeit unbeknownst to himself. Similarly, Thucydides' Athenian plague is seen right after the death of Pericles, arguably the high point in the work, and the history of Athens. Pericles had similarly warned the Athenians against expanding their empire and keeping their greed in check. In all these three instances, it seems probable that the authors are trying to propagate certain reasons for the onslaught of the plague, thereby rationalizing the plague's onset upon the people.

It is only in the medical writings of Hippocrates, that we see a description of the plague which is removed from any moral didactic teleology perpetrated by its describers. By using the term *epidemios*, Hippocrates suggests that the disease is merely symptoms shared by everyone, similar to ideas and customs shared by everyone in the community. The point to reiterate is that Hippocrates never associated a negative connotation with this shared ailment of the body, nor did he equate it with the moral or mental corruption of the masses. *Epidemios*, in the Hippocratic sense, almost has a euphemistic quality to describe the burden of disease. This burden, by being circulated in and across the masses, is alleviated from being the consequences of one's own actions to an accident whose etiology cannot be known but can be treated and healed.

While in hindsight it is easy, perhaps obvious, for us to see how the term *epidemios* replaced the earlier nomenclatures of *nosos* and *loimos*, it would probably have been an absurd suggestion for the average Athenian. Hindsight is a privilege that we have only when examining the posteriority (Roese and Vohs, 2012, pp. 411–426). The consequences of the Athenian plague manifested themselves, in socio-religious aspects by establishing the cult of Asclepius, to be built adjacent to every theater. Whereas the enhanced understanding of the human body and its afflictions with diseases manifested themselves in language by abandoning the usage of terms that carried negative connotations. Instead, it is euphemized in an existing, similar term with a positive, and hopeful ring to it. The modern equivalent of this phenomenon can be seen in the evolutionary naming of the HIV disease. The earlier signifiers for the ailment constituted terms such as "gay plague, gay disease, and GRID or Gay related immune deficiency" (Burridge and Benczes, 2018, p. 38). Apart from being explicitly offensive on a number of tangents, these labels directly placed the blame for contracting the disease on the grounds of having a certain sexual lifestyle (Treichler, 1987, p. 31). These terms were eventually dropped for the contemporary term "aids," now used to describe the symptoms of the virus. The term AIDS, apart from being inclusive, has a particularly positive ring to it since the word also means "to help." The language change in these cases was marked by a composite number of reasons that censored or tabooed the earlier forms of language on social, religious, and psychological grounds.

Ultimately, the spreading, evolving, and ever-morphing nature of language is much akin to that of a disease, forever spreading, and evolving. There are ways in which we can specify language change as categorical, rational, and predictable, just as we can do for diseases and plagues. Yet sometimes this process is irrational, illogical, and unpredictable. Both of them can either be described as a blanket of all-encompassing, non-discriminating shadow that consumes all in its wake; or a systematic network of mazes that boroughs through the annals of history, a method in madness, or perhaps none at all.

Bibliography

Anthony, D.W., et al. (1986) The 'Kurgan Culture', Indo-European Origins, and the Domestication of the Horse: A Reconsideration. *Current Anthropology*, 27(4), pp. 291–313.

Bernheim, F and Zener, A. A. (1978) The Sminthian Apollo and the Epidemic among the Achaeans at Troy. *Transactions of the American Philological Association (1974-)*, 108, pp. 11–14.

Burridge, K. and Allan, K. (2007) *Forbidden Words: Taboo and the Censoring of Language*, Cambridge University Press.

Burridge, K. and Benczes, R.A. (2018) Speaking of disease and death. In: K. Allan (ed.) *The Oxford Handbook of Taboo Words and Language*. Oxford University Press, pp. 61–77. https://doi.org/10.1093/oxfordhb/9780198808190.013.4

Emeneau, M.B. (1948) Taboos on Animal Names. *Language*, 24(1), pp. 57. https://doi.org/10.2307/410287

Feldman, H. (1959) The Problem of Personal Names as a Universal Element in Culture. *American Imago*, 16, 3, p. 237. http://www.jstor.org/stable/26301715

Foucault, M. (1988) *Madness and Civilization: A History of Insanity in the Age of Reason*. New York: New York Random House.

Girard, R. (1974) The Plague in Literature and Myth. *Texas Studies in Literature and Language*, 15(5), pp. 833–850.

Grimm, J. and Wilhelm, G. (1904) *Grimm's Fairy Tales*. Edited by J.H. Fassett. New York: The Macmillan Company; London: Macmillan & Co., Ltd.

Guvendir, E. (2015) Why are Males Inclined to Use Strong Swear Words More Than Females? An Evolutionary Explanation Based on Male Intergroup Aggressiveness. *Language Sciences*, 50, pp. 133–139.

Heath, J.G. (1984) Language Contact and Language Change. *Annual Review of Anthropology*, 13, pp. 367–384.

Hock, H. (1986) *Principles of Historical Linguistics*. Berlin, Boston: De Gruyter Mouton, pp. 34–51.

Homer (1919) *The Odyssey: in Two Volumes*. 2. Translated by A.T. Murray. Massachusetts: Harvard University Press.

Homer (1924) *The Iliad*. Translated by A.T. Murray. London: W. Heinemann; New York: G.P. Putnam's Sons.

Leben, W.R. (2018) *Languages of the World. Oxford Research Encyclopedia of Linguistics*. Oxford: Oxford University Press, p 1.

Leglise, I. and Migge, B. (2006) Language-Naming Practices, Ideologies, and Linguistic Practices: Toward a Comprehensive Description of Language Varieties. *Language in Society*, 35(3), pp. 313–339. https://doi.org/10.1017/S0047404506060155

Lehmann, W.P. (1992) *Historical Linguistics: An Introduction*. London: Routledge.
Lehmann, W.P. (2008) Linguistic Laws and Universals: The Twain. In: H.H. Hock (ed.) *Studies in Slavic and General Linguistics*. Berlin, Boston: De Gruyter Mouton, pp. 32–34.
Littman, R.J. (2009) The Plague of Athens: Epidemiology and Paleopathology. *Mount Sinai Journal of Medicine*, 76, pp. 456–467.
Lloyd, G.E.R. (2003) *In the Grip of Disease: Studies in the Greek Imagination*. Oxford: Oxford University Press.
Mallory, J.P. and Adams, D.Q. (1997) *Encyclopedia of Indo-European Culture*. London: Fitzroy Dearborn.
Mallory, J.P. and Adams, D.Q. (2006) *The Oxford Introduction to Proto-Indo-European and the Proto-Indo-European World (Oxford Linguistics)*. Oxford: Oxford University Press.
Marquis, A.G. (1978) Words as Weapons: Propaganda in Britain and Germany during the First World War. *Journal of Contemporary History*, 13(3), pp. 467–498.
Martin, P.M.V. and Martin-Granel, E. (2006) 2,500-Year Evolution of the Term Epidemic. *Emerging Infectious Diseases*, 12(6), p. 977. https://doi.org/10.3201/eid1206.051263
Mitchell-Boyask, R. (2008) *Plague and the Athenian Imagination: Drama, History and the cult of Asclepius*. Cambridge: Cambridge University Press.
Nelkin, D. and Gilman, S.L. (1988) Placing Blame for Devastating Disease. *Social Research*, 55(3), pp. 361–378.
Page, D.L. (1953) Thucydides' Description of the Great Plague at Athens. *The Classical Quarterly*, 3(3/4), pp. 97–119.
Rissanen, M. (2008) From 'Quickly' to 'Fairly': On the History of Rather. *English Language and Linguistics*, 12(02), 345–359. https://doi.org/10.1017/S1360674308002657
Roese, N.J. and Vohs, K.D. (2012) Hindsight bias. *Perspectives on Psychological Science*, 7(5), pp. 411–426.
Sokal, R.R., et al. (1992) Origins of the Indo-Europeans: Genetic Evidence. *Proceedings of the National Academy of Sciences of the United States of America*, 89(16), pp. 7669–7673.
Sophocles (1887) *Oedipus Tyrannus*. Translated by R. Webb. Cambridge: Cambridge University Press.
Thucydides (1910) *The Peloponnesian War*. Translated by R. Crawley. Perseus Digital Library.
Treichler, P.A., (1987) AIDS, Homophobia, and Biomedical Discourse: An Epidemic of Signification. *October*, 43, pp. 31–70.

5

"MY RACE IS NOT MY VIRUS"

Affective Racial Algorithms during Covid-19 Pandemic

Sayan Parial

Human civilization from its genesis has been facing moments of transition, exchange, and transformation. The catastrophic phenomenon of Covid-19 pandemic had been such a moment of transition in human history that would never let humanity escape from its affective imprints upon the collective human psyche. Having said that, under the collective umbrella of this humanitarian crisis lies numerous narratives and responses to similar crises from different communities belonging to different social and geo-political spaces. Hence, these multiple expressions and meanings demand critical inquiry to unfold the narratives and responses of the Covid-19 pandemic.

The Covid-19 pandemic is not only a bio-medical crisis, but it also brought in a sea change in the way we used to think of the politics of care, protection, and, most importantly, perception. This chapter, thus, attempts to expose the failure of neo-liberal care of neo-capitalist states amid the pandemic by unmasking how their political and media machinery, digital affordances, and algorithms are being circulated by news agencies within the Western countries to form an exclusionary perception to systematically stigmatize the non-white communities and trigger age-old racial scars. This chapter, thus, also hinges on how democratic values are being thwarted by the consolidation and amplification of xenophobia and racial disparities in the West during Covid-19 pandemic. It addresses how the systemic circulation of the naming of the Delta variant of coronavirus as "Indian variant," "Chinese virus," or "African variant", and so on in the West through different media platforms and, even, by the institutional bodies of the Western countries is creating a xenophobic atmosphere and destabilizing the existential certainty of non-whites. These discriminatory representations of the non-whites

DOI: 10.4324/9781003590392-8

have caused semantic racial prejudices against the Asian, African, and South Asian diasporic communities residing there. This nomenclature of the virus with the geographical label has unleashed a series of marketed and capitalized transversal "affects" to sustain power relations. This chapter, bringing insights from the philosophy of "affect," aims to study the Western media reporting during the pandemic and to trace the assemblages of mass media, and institutional actors in a network of exchange that formulates a certain kind of racial rhetoric for intensifying a collective suspicion among the whites, and a sense of alienation among the non-whites in the West. So, this media-generated affective "stickiness" or attachments among signs, bodies, and objects as an outcome of a fusion of racial capitalism and environmental injustice is re-territorializing the members of diasporic communities at the margins by mathematizing them to be controlled by socio-political machinery of the institutions of power.

The naming of the virus in the name of geographic location can unleash severe repercussions. It can create agitation and suspicion among the masses and lead to racism, and xenophobia, and can also impose stigma upon the people. For instance, former president Donald Trump labeled the coronavirus as the "Chinese virus," which inflamed a certain amount of hatred from the American people against the Asian communities living in America. Language works in multiple layers; thus, it needs to be employed with concern and care since unethical or unparliamentary comments can lead to dire consequences. The naming of the virus as the "Chinese virus" triggered a dramatic growth in racial slurs and physical violence against Asian Americans.

There are several other instances as well that show the proliferation of racial slang by the white community to the non-whites. Rohini Mohan (2021), in *The Straits Times*, writes about such instances, like, a Caucasian patient infected by the virus denies being treated by a doctor of an East or South Asian origin and demands a different doctor of Western origin. An Indian doctor working in a Texas hospital during the pandemic said that he had never been conscious about his ethnicity in his whole working life. Still, during the pandemic, his ethnicity became a barrier to treating white patients. After naming the B1617 strain of the virus as the "Indian Variant", the people living in the United States, Britain, Australia, Singapore, and elsewhere started feeling a sense of alienation and anxiety in the countries they had been residing for several years. Mr Indrajit Veerakumar, an oil rig operator in Singapore, said that he found himself in desperation to return to his homeland Tamil Nadu as the quarantine rules and "dirty looks" from the people were imposing a tag of "virus carriers" upon the patients of Covid. A senior executive of a software company from Sydney said that his colleagues started taking "a step back" from her because of the suspicion amid the atmosphere in the West regarding Indians. Even during a match between India and England at Trent Bridge, the English fans kept shouting the term "delta" to humiliate the Indian fans and, even, the Indian players who were fielding near the boundary (Anjum, 2021). According to the Stop AAIP Hate report, 3,795 racist attacks on Asian Americans have been reported between March 19, 2020, and February 28, 2021, out of which 11.1% of cases are of physical assaults (Reinstein, 2021). New York-based publication house *The Juggernaut* also pointed out that WhatsApp and Facebook messages are being disseminated in the United States blaming the Asian communities for the spread of the infectious variant of the virus (Sur, 2021). On April 22, the newspaper *Journal de Montreal* published the image of the Canadian Prime Minister wearing Indian clothes on their front page and the headline was "the variant from India has arrived" in French, which was a direct racist attack against the Indian community or Asian community, following which the newspaper had to publish an apology (Prakash, 2021). To get rid of this precarious condition, the Indian ministry had requested to remove posts with the caption "Indian Variant" from social media platforms. WHO also decided to rename the virus' strains with scientific names such as alpha, delta, beta, and gamma as naming the virus with connection to the geographical space of origin can form anti-immigrant, white supremacist, ultra-nationalist, and xenophobic conspiracy theories that may criminalize refugees and foreigners. Due to such a topsy-turvy situation, the World Health Organization tweeted:

> WHO does not identify viruses or variants with names of countries they are first reported from. We refer to them by their scientific names and request all to do the same for consistency.
>
> *(WHO, 2021)*

In their tweet, they tagged the Press Information Bureau and several leading Indian media houses. Hours after WHO tweeted, *The Washington Post* headline was "Indian Coronavirus variant has now spread to almost 50 countries, says WHO", and *The New York Times* headline was "Covid-19: W.H.O. Warns India's Homegrown Virus Variant May Be Highly Contagious" (Singh, 2021). *The Times* even used the "Indian variant" in their headline in an article, the *Daily Mail* also referred to "Indian variant hotspots" in a headline, and the BBC published an article headlined, "Covid: Indian variant 'now dominant' in the UK," at the start of June (Ireland, 2021). The article refers to the variant as Delta, but the question is why "Indian Variant" is used in the title. These headlines contradict the tweets of WHO regarding the naming of the virus. The General Secretary of the UN, António Guterres, warned:

> Covid-19 does not care who we are, where we live, what we believe or about any other distinction. We need every ounce of solidarity to tackle it together. Yet the pandemic continues to unleash a tsunami of hate and xenophobia, scapegoating and scare-mongering.
>
> *(UN Peace and Security, 2020)*

Certain tag lines, titles, and slurring are intentionally being brought into the discourse to disseminate a colonial ideology under the shadow of an impartial and neutral enterprise of the Western media houses. These strategies are ideologically designed by interlinked mechanisms of power with a motive to dehumanize, derogate, or derecognize, a certain targeted section of the populace for disempowering the minority or the people of/from the margins and also for imposing a negative stereotype upon the targeted community. Aimé Césaire once said, "The commonest curse is to be the dupe in good faith of a collective hypocrisy that cleverly misrepresents problems, the better to legitimize the hateful solutions provided by them" (Césaire, 2000, p. 2). So, this "collective hypocrisy" of the institutions of state and media houses of the West is legitimizing such racial misrepresentations to devalue, degrade, and defame the non-white communities. Such discriminatory practices manufacture a hierarchy in society by infusing "strangeness" and alienation for the non-whites within Western countries. This whole phenomenon of blaming, and targeting, the minority in times of crisis also showcases the specter of racism, which still haunts humanity. This stereotypical mindset gets solidified in global politics and popular imagination, and consolidated in the socio-political cultural and economic domains of knowledge. Print or online media creates an anti-Asian or anti-African perception in the collective consciousness of the West by systematically misrepresenting different phenomena and normalizing the hegemonic structure of the society.

As an outcome of the xenophobic atmosphere, several digital campaigns were launched by the Asian and African communities to unleash a counter-narrative to the prejudiced and homogenized perception of the whites about the non-whites. The social media campaigns like "#IamNotaVirus", the Black Lives Matter movement, and so on were raising ethical-racial awareness concerning ethno-racial discrimination in general. However, the attacks only increased and reached their peak in the United States after the murder of six Asian descendants in Atlanta a year after the outbreak of the virus (Nicole and Jonah, 2021).

During the Covid-19 pandemic, when the public was increasingly involved in several digital platforms, the circulation of numerous racial algorithms accelerated a mass consumption of anti-black rhetoric. In the digital age, algorithms are popular and effective equipment often employed by different governmental and non-governmental organizations to propagate their ideologies and separatist politics to maintain limited transparency and accountability. Many political thinkers and media theorists have engaged in the exercise of employing algorithms in today's digital world and observed the vulnerable side of algorithms that can fracture the collective perception of a community. Algorithmic bias may deteriorate into algorithmic injustice. Algorithmic Injustice works in a networked reality. There is a chain of events associated with it. The crisis of the pandemic was weaponized by the different institutions of media and the state to criminalize the people of color living in the West. The algorithms during the time of Covid-19 became the mediums for imparting racial discriminatory ideology in the minds of the people. So, the period of struggle during this health crisis went to the extremes for the Asians and the Africans when the whole socio-political system started blaming the people of color for the outbreak of the virus. Hence, their racial identity started haunting them like a virus during this crisis. Although algorithms thrive because of their agency to trace the needs and preferences of individuals, the media ecosystem may use the algorithms to, even, threaten democratic communication by reinforcing fractured and politically motivated worldviews and partial information. Algorithms focus on the maximization of the engagement of the consumers who see content in social media, consume it, and then share it and reshare it to different platforms. Once the content is formed, it reaches a larger audience with a chain reaction. As the viewers' count increases, it gradually gets viral and creates a collective preference, which often bends the reality and fabricates a bias among the consumers regarding any particular phenomenon of society.

These algorithms divide individuals into numerous pieces based on their ethnicity, religion, color, desires, dislikes, doings in social media, etc. The media houses are utilizing this fragmented nature of individuality to control the consumers on a cognitive scale. Deleuze and Guattari (1994) has pointed out that because of this fragmented reality of individuality, individuals become "dividuals." In his brief essay, "Postscript on the Societies of Control", Deleuze shows how technologies control individuals. He extends Michel Foucault's work *Discipline and Punish* (1977) to trace these new technologies of control. These new control technologies divide individuals into dividuals and form "societies of control," which is an extension of Michel Foucault's "Disciplinary Societies." The media-generated affective relationality among signs, bodies, and objects reshapes human perception and forms a marketed consciousness to accelerate mass consumption. Racial slurs, social media memes, and tweets by the political delegates are being weaponized to disseminate a particular ideology of hatred among the Western populace. Such separatist ideology is employed to homogenize the society and distract the citizens from the burning issues related to their well-being. These media operations are creating precarious conditions for minority communities. This socio-political precarity within a bio-medical crisis creates an atmosphere of racial capitalism and environmental injustice since human subjects are being mathematized by inscribing them with codes, media-generated algorithms, and so on to form docile bodies to be controlled. The intention to reconstruct the biological self incorporating digital data sets forms fragmented human identities and perceptions. Thus, the self loses control over their own perception and identity. The self because of this new form of racial subjugation lives with its unknown digital other. This "other" influences the self's perception and thinkability unconsciously. Hence, the individual is a connected whole; in other words, the individual is no individual since the very individuality is divided and fragmented. The individuals according to Deleuze (1992, p. 5) are "dividuals" to be controlled and manipulated by fluid interactions between institutions of power. "Dividual"—a physically embodied human subject that is divisible and reducible to data sets through different institutional bodies or other organizations. Deleuze coined the term "dividual" to talk about the mechanisms of "societies of control." The term "individual" means indivisible. But at the micro-political level, human subjects can be seen as a divided actant because of their associativeness with heterogeneous socio-political, cultural, and technological apparatuses.

So, these racial algorithms, nomenclatures based on geography, news headlines, etc., circulate affects through media agencies, which influence human consumers' judgments, behaviors, attitudes, and perceptions toward something. Media theories show the mimetic nature of the media-generated affects has a close inclination with Aristotle's understanding of mimesis, as in *Poetics*, Aristotle argues that a perfect tragedy should imitate actions that can excite "pity and fear" (Daniels and Scully, 1992, p. 204). The ability to excite or influence is the salient feature of affect. Baruch Spinoza also offers valuable thoughts on affect in his work *Ethics*. He defines affect as "the modifications of the body whereby the active power of the said body is increased or diminished"

(Spinoza, 1955, p. 130). Spinoza puts emphasis on the modifications of the human body, which shows how affect is pre-personal and goes beyond the control of the body. All human activity, including cognition, produces and is produced by affect. In *Matter and Memory*, Henri Bergson (2004, p. 60) finds a correlation between cognition and affect as he observes affect is "part or aspect of the inside of our bodies which mix with the image of external bodies." This "part or aspect" produces our perception, our worldview as in the words of Bergson there is no perception without affection (Bergson, 2004, p. 60). In *What Is Philosophy* (1994), Felix Guattari and Gilles Deleuze (1994, p. 163) talk about how aesthetics unleashes a sense of affect as the oeuvre of aesthetics is "a bloc of sensations, that is to say, a compound of percepts and affects." The discursive formulation of affect is bringing different disciplines of thoughts into an epistemic space where the affect is being studied as something embodied in the human consciousness and interrelated to human cognition. Marshall McLuhan (1994, p. 8), a media theorist, also links affect to the media studies as he finds each media is marked by "the change of scale or pace or pattern that it introduces into human affairs." The above discussion propounds the agential quality and multiplicity of affect as it engages with human cognition, influences it, and reformulates it. It is not an isolated agential entity; rather, "[i]t's an event, or a dimension of every event" (Loktev and Massumi, 2008, p. 183). The media houses in the West through the naming of the virus as the Indian variant have unleashed a series of affective shocks, more specifically, micro-shocks, which are interrelated to the effect of affect. The micro-shocks are micro not because they are "micro" in their degree of affectability; rather, here micro means the workings of affect, which are very hard to document rationally since it is diversly networked and beyond the apparent cognition. The affectability of the affects had the faculty of invisibility, which works through multiple pathways. This is also the nature of ideology that creates an illusion of reality in front of us and then affects us. The socio-political Eurocentric narrative-driven ideologies in different media platforms are intervening in the consumers' consciousness and forming perceptions in their minds. They are consuming these materials, which implicitly formulate micro-perceptions through shock formation. We are always in a space populated with shocks, more specifically micro-shocks that often pass away even without knocking our consciousness as it only registers in their effects. These micro-shocks are relatable to the micro-perceptions, which are not small perceptions; rather, they are virtual in nature that the body cannot grab at its first impact. It brings the selves, with its many differential potentialities, into a transitory phase of becoming. The consumers of the news are forming within themselves a shared hatred for the non-whites and sometimes these beliefs are converting into actions, reactions, and agitations. When we act, we are actualizing the affectability of affect in practice. The racial hatred during Covid-19 is the actualization of the media-driven affective ideologies. But affects work differently for different individuals. So, the racial slurring through articles, algorithms, and social media posts is on the one hand inflaming anger and aggressive xenophobic attitudes in some people of the West and leading them toward agitation and on the other hand forming fear and anxiety in those who are of Asian or African origin. These agitations and reactions give life to the ghost of the colonial past even in today's world. This past is a very active past that is reappearing and repeating itself through these "oppressive slurs" in moments of crisis.

Slurring can be seen as a neocolonial activity that is motivated by hegemonic essentialism and reductionism. This neocolonialism is, according to Philip Altbach (1971, p. 237), "a planned policy of advanced nations to maintain their influence in developing countries." Slurs manufacture a fortress of unjust power imbalance through "role assignment." Roles are, according to Goffman (1972, p. 75), the foci of socialization, since society imposes particular roles for specific social performance. Social roles participate in structuring social interactionism and the discursive status and roles of individuals or groups. These words can also initiate violent action, as Tirrell observes (2012, p. 174), that derogative words are "action-engendering" and "can be part and parcel of genocide, not only an antecedent of it."

Slur is just not only a term or word; rather, it is an action in itself that works with an implied ideology. The ideology behind the slurs is unleashed with a desire to convert the individual into a subject of hatred. This conscious conversion from individual to subject is similar to the notion of Louis Althusser's notion of "Interpellation." As he said:

> I ... suggest that ideology 'acts' or 'functions' in such a way that it 'recruits' subjects among the individuals ... or 'transforms' the individuals into subjects ... by that very precise operation which I have called interpellation or hailing, and which can be imagined along the lines of the most commonplace everyday ... hailing: 'Hey, you there!' The hailed individual will turn round. By this mere one-hundred and-eighty-degree physical conversion, he becomes a subject. Why? Because he has recognized that the hail was 'really' addressed to him, and that 'it was really' him who was hailed (and not someone else).
>
> *(Althusser, 1971, p. 174)*

Derek Hook coins the phrase "technology of affect" to show how Western media forms interpellated subjects and intensifies the affective stereotypes, and, thus, with the repetitive stereotypical images perpetuates an "ineradicable distinction between Western superiority and Oriental inferiority" (Al-'Azm, 2010, p. 55). Technology includes an assemblage of discourses, practices, knowledge, and techniques. As Hook observes:

> [E]xpert system comprised of a discrete set of [...] applied knowledges and/or forms of specialist language, which is used by experts on deviant subjects [...] as means of achieving a productive output of sorts, a relation of greater mastery or control.
>
> *(Hook, 2005, p. 9)*

These stereotypes with their affective dissemination and repetitive reappearances hamper the existing social symmetry. Sabiha Allouche observes (2015, p. 128) in her work on the technology of affects that a "stereotype affects one's relationality with others and triggers negative attachments, such as racism or homophobia, which become increasingly enacted on the surface." These slurs have a refrain-like quality, as Deleuze observes (1987, p. 317), that a refrain is "rhythm and melody that have been territorialized because they have become expressive because they are territorializing." It is affective because of its territorializing nature and its agency to regulate the society. The collaboration between the Western media and foreign policies is institutionalizing the notion of strangeness in the Asian community. The ideology of hatred was actualized by the repetitive refrain-like articulation of racial rhetoric through different media platforms.

Affects are sticky attachments, as Sara Ahmed says (2004, p. 92), "A stereotype occupies a territory of impressions that is maintained by a power structure that allows it to proliferate and to 'stick' to the point it operates as affect." Even though structural imbalance through the formulation of affective stickiness is acknowledged, European countries neglect these aspects of the legitimized network of racism that breaks the ethical structure of the society. Hate consolidates power in a neocolonial structure and perpetuates exploitation. Racism, as Kendi offered (2019, p. 17), "is a marriage of racist policies and racist ideas that produce and normalize racial inequalities ..." During this pandemic, a considerable number of Western Media houses worked through certain frameworks to normalize hatred and disseminate a particular agenda among the commoners to perpetuate racial stereotypes and bring focus on the compartmentalized Asian and African communities residing in America or any other European countries. Framing theory of media studies shows how the Western media houses were active in including and excluding certain words, images, concepts, and information to affect people's perceptions and initiate politically motivated actions. Covid-19 as an event or phenomenon witnessed how, in a situation of crisis, humanity reacts, and how the notion of existence becomes politically contested. The Western media reporting foreign policies of the state and the racial disparities during the pandemic show how every phenomenon is in a network of association between language, human body, race, ethnicity, colonial education, institution, and policies, and how they all are coexisting together, intra-acting and interacting with each other reconstructing knowledge, deconstructing structures, forming perceptions, realities, affecting others, and in the process get affected. Hence, the pandemic, which is apparently a bio-medical crisis, becomes a double threat for certain communities because of their ethnic identity with affective shocks circulated through media and state-driven racial stereotypes, even, in an age where the Western neo-liberal states are extolling the notions of care and hospitality.

Bibliography

Ahmed, S. (2004) *The Cultural Politics of Emotion*. New York: Routledge.

Al-'Azm, S. J. (2010) Orientalism and Orientalism in Reverse. In: G. Ritzer and Z. Atalay (eds.) *Readings in Globalisation: Key Concepts and Major Debates*. Chichester: Blackwell Publishing Ltd, pp. 54–56.

Allouche, S. (2015) Western Media as 'Technology of Affect': The Affective Making of the Angry Young Man. *Graduate Journal of Social Science*, *11*(1), pp. 120–142.

Altbach, P.G. (1971) Education and Neocolonialism: A Note. *Comparative Education Review*, 15(2), pp. 237–239.

Althusser, L. (1971) Ideology and Ideological State Apparatuses. In: L. Althusser (ed.) *Lenin and Philosophy*. New York: Monthly Review Press, pp. 127–186.

Ananny, M. and Crawford, K. (2016) Seeing Without Knowing: Limitations of the Transparency Ideal and Its Application to Algorithmic Accountability. *New Media & Society*, 20(3), pp. 973–989.

Anjum, S. (2021) ENG v IND 2021: English Fans Kept Chanting 'Delta' – British Indian Woman Claims Copping Racial Abuse at Trent Bridge. [Online] *Circle of Cricket*. Available at: https://circleofcricket.com/category/engvind2021/67973/eng-v-ind-2021-english-fanskept-chanting-delta-british-indian-woman-claims-copping-racial-abuse-at-trent-bridge (Accessed: 7 May, 2023).

Bergson, H. (2004) *Matter and Memory*. New York: Dover Publications.
Césaire, A. (2000) *Discourse on Colonialism*. Translated by J. Pinkham. New York: Monthly Review Press.
Daniels, C.B. and Scully, S. (1992) Pity, Fear, and Catharsis in Aristotle's Poetics. *Noûs*, 26(2), pp. 204–217.
Deleuze, G. (1992) Postscript on the Societies of Control. *October*, 59, pp. 3–7.
Deleuze, G. and Guattari, F. (1987) *A Thousand Plateaus: Capitalism and Schizophrenia*. Translated by B. Massumi. Minneapolis: University of Minnesota Press.
Deleuze, G. and Guattari, F. (1994) *What Is Philosophy*. Translated by H. Tomlinson and G. Burchell. New York: Columbia University Press.
Foucault, M. (1977) *Discipline and Punish: The Birth of the Prison*. New York: Pantheon Books.
Goffman, E. (1972) *Encounters: Two studies in the Sociology of Interaction*. England: Penguin.
Hook, D. (2005) Affecting Whiteness: Racism as Technology of Affect. *International Journal of Critical Psychology*, 16, pp. 74–99. Available at: http://eprints.lse.ac.uk/archive/00000956 (Accessed: 28 September, 2014).
Ireland, E. (2021) The WHO Says That the New COVID Variant Should Be Referred to as the "Delta Variant". So Why Are Newspapers Still Calling It the "Indian" Variant? [Online] *Hacked Off*. Available at: https://hackinginquiry.org/the-who-says-that-the-new-covid-variant-should-be-referrd-to-as-the-delta-variant-so-why-are-newspapers-still-calling-it-the-indian-variant/ (Accessed: 7 May, 2023).
Kendi, I.X. (2019) *How to Be an Anti-Racist*. New York: Penguin Random House.
Loktev, J. and Massumi, B. (2008) Of Microperception and Micropolitics: An Interview with Brian Massumi, 15 August. *Inflexions*, 3, pp. 183–275.
McLuhan, M. (1994) *Understanding Media: The Extensions of Man*. Massachusetts: The MIT Press.
Mohan, R. (2021) Overseas Indians Hope Renaming of Covid-19 Variants Will Reduce Stigma. [Online] *The Straits Time*. Available at: https://www.straitstimes.com/asia/south-asia/overseas-indians-hope-renaming-of-cornavirus-variants-will-reduce-stigma (Accessed: 7 May, 2023).
Nicole, H. and Jonah, B. (2021) Asian-Americans Are Being Attacked. Why Are Hate Crime Charges So Rare. [Online] *New York Times*. Available at: https://www.nytimes.com/2021/03/18/nyregion/asian-hate-crimes.html (Accessed: 7 May, 2023).
Prakash, P. (2021) Global Spread of Covid-19 Variant First Detected in India Brings with It Fears of Anti-Indian Racism. [Online] *Scroll*. Available at: https://scroll.in/global/995805/global-spread-of-covid-19-variant-first-detected-in-inda-brings-with-it-fears-of-anti-indian-racism#:~:text=From%20Singapore%20to%20te%20US%20to%20

Australia%2C%20incidents%20of%20anti,1.617%20variant.&tet=Reuters%2FShannon%20Stapleton-,The%20B.,53%20countries%20around%20th%20world (Accessed: 7 May, 2023).
Reinstein, J. (2021) There Have Been At Least 3,795 Hate Incidents Against Asian Americans During The Pandemic, A New Report Shows. [Online] *BuzzFeed*. Available at: https://www.buzzfeednews.com/article/juliareinstein/anti-asian-racist-hate-incidents (Accessed: 7 May, 2023).
Singh, S. (2021) Why Calling the Covid B.1.617 Strain Indian Variant Reeks of Agenda. [Online] *DailyO*. Available at: https://www.dailyo.in/variety/covid-19-b-1-617-indian-variant-western-media-racism34567 (Accessed: 7 May, 2023).
Spinoza, B. (1955) *Works of Spinoza V. II*. Translated by R.H.M. Elwes. New York: Dover Publications.
Sur, S. (2021) "Be Careful": WhatsApp Forwards Spread Fear and Misinformation. [Online] *The Juggernaut*. Available at: https://www.jgnt.co/whatsapp-forwards-stoke-fear-and-spread-misinformation-durin-india-covid-crisis (Accessed: 7 May, 2023).
Tirrell, L. (2012). Genocidal Language Games. In: I. Maitra and M.K. McGowan (eds.), *Speech and Harm: Controversies Over Free Speech*. Oxford: Oxford University Press, pp. 174–221.
UN Peace and Security. (2020) UN Chief Appeals for Global Action Against Coronavirus-Fueled Hate Speech. [Online] Available at: https://operationalsupport.un.org/en/un-chief-appeals-global-action-against-coronavirus-fueled-hate-speech (Accessed: 7 May, 2023).
WHO. (2021) WHO Does Not Identify Viruses or Variants with Names of Countries. *Twitter*, [Online] 12 May. Available at: https://x.com/WHOSEARO/status/1392396456774955014 (Accessed: 7 May, 2023).

6

DEATHLY GAMES

Playing in the Pandemic

Gaurav Kumar

A story on *The Times of India's* website from March 27, 2020, takes us right back to the onset of the Covid-19 pandemic in many parts of the world. "Why would anyone want to lick toilet seats?", the article begins by asking and answers it by explaining that it was part of a trend on the social media app TikTok called the Coronavirus challenge, which "started after content creator Ava Louise did a video to prove that it was perfectly alright (sic) to lick the toilets eat inside an airplane bathroom to become 'viral' on TikTok" (*The Times of India*, 2020). Many suspected those participating in the challenge often faked their participation using edited pictures/texts and sometimes the subsequent illnesses caused by the act just for the attention such acts garner. One of the participants partially confirmed the hypothesis by announcing to a reporter that "I was tired of that b—h corona getting more publicity than ME. I'm the real celebrity." Are the participants of this challenge really facing up to the arrival of a new, scary virus and challenging the unsettling possibility of death that it entailed for many of us in early 2020? That would hardly be true if we go by the conventional meaning of a challenge, especially a challenge on TikTok. The Cambridge Dictionary defines "challenge" as "the situation of being faced with) something that needs great mental or physical effort in order to be done successfully and therefore tests a person's ability" but also as "an invitation to compete or take part, especially in a game or argument." A game implies that the activities you participate in as part of the game are in some way removed from the real, everyday world and, therefore, not subject to many of its rules, causalities, and events, including, hopefully, the event of death, which is to be mastered through such death-defying stunts. Moreover, the configuration of such challenges on social media websites/apps achieved using hashtags and viral news articles clearly

DOI: 10.4324/9781003590392-9

promises the assurance of the participant's fame for posterity, which is, in fact, the motivation for undertaking such challenges. In other words, the participant is convinced that he will live on—as a viral video/image/profile or a living, breathing champion—irrespective of the outcome of the challenge. This is the opposite of grasping death seriously and philosophically, very different from staring at the actual possibility of death, which implies reflecting on the absolute annihilation of one's existence and the nothingness that would ensue.

A similar catachresis, couched in idioms of bravery and martyrdom, can be traced in many cultures that valorize the martyrdom of their heroes. Janet Kamphorst's book *In Praise of Death: History and Poetry in Medieval Marwar* (2008), for instance, tracks the "warlike poetry" and "martial ethos" of medieval Rajasthani heroic and epic poetry, which often focuses on the "deification of warriors" through martyrdom, an act that proved their allegiance to *Dharma* in bravely facing death, ensuring them a place in heaven as well as literature, life, and culture of the posterity (p. 11). Kamphorst tells us:

> By describing how blood gushes in battle, lives are taken, warriors are beheaded but their torsos continue to fight, attention is called to the fact that Pabuji, Jimda and their warriors do not fear death but, on the contrary, seek it out eagerly.
>
> *(p. 125)*

However, if the goal of such literature is to negate and overcome the fear of death by translating it as an embrace of the heavenly/futurity, it is an act of mistranslation of the ontology of death that is shared by such religions or thought systems across the world as they offer the prospect of another world or heaven as continuity of and compensation for death, in effect declawing its existential serrations. This chapter intends to look at some other ways of denying or "playing" with death—in the form of social media challenges or defiant partying—in an attempt to understand our reactions to the Covid-19 pandemic and the confrontation of death it entailed for many of us who lived and died during this pandemic.

Both the acts of dalliance with death mentioned above seem to constitute what Irvin D. Yalom (2008) calls denial of death (anxiety). In *Staring at the Sun: Overcoming the Terror of Death* (2008), he makes the claim that the awareness and trauma of our mortality—the realization that we will certainly die at some point to return to "dust" or nothingness—overshadows all human existence. It may manifest "as generalized unrest"/"another psychological symptom" or as an "explicit and conscious stream of anxiety about death" (p. 2). He quotes Epicurus to make the claim that death anxiety "interferes with one's enjoyment of life and leaves no pleasure undisturbed" (p. 3). In early childhood, children observing deaths around them learn to wonder but stay silent apropos the topic by imitating their parents, who often try to provide reassurance and comfort when interrogated by offering distractions, or by pushing death into the distant future or by discussing the resurrection, union, and eternity promised by most religions or belief systems. Cyclical phases of forgetting and returning follow this phase of life. Adolescents, since they are at the threshold of a new life, think a lot about beginnings and endings (witness, says Yalom, regular spurts in suicides among the teenage population) and try to master death through their life projects, artworks, or games (e.g., video games/adventures/activities that seem to make them "masters and dispensers of death," horror movies, songs, and memes about death). This preoccupation with life and death may be pushed aside by concerns related to career and family as we grow into adults but usually returns with what is termed a "midlife crisis," wherein we try to make sense of the trajectory and meaning of our lives (and deaths). This cyclicity is a good thing, says Yalom, for

> It's not easy to live every moment wholly aware of death. It's like trying to stare the sun in the face: you can stand only so much of it. Because we cannot live frozen in fear, we generate methods to soften death's terror. We project ourselves into the future through our children; we grow rich, famous, ever larger; we develop compulsive protective rituals; or we embrace an impregnable belief in an ultimate rescuer.
>
> *(p. 5)*

One of the most common sites for achieving this denial of death, says Yalom, is religion itself, which "not only softens the pain of mortality through some vision of everlasting life but also palliates fearful isolation by offering an eternal presence, and provides a clear blueprint for living a meaningful life" (p. 5). Yalom's goal is to provide a philosophical account of an existentialist therapy that considers many symptoms and behaviors, such as anxiety or depression, obsessive attachments to a cause or community, or states, such as obsessive promiscuity on dating apps as our refusal to come to terms with the painful confrontation with the possibility of our non-being. He goes so far as to say that "one could argue that the psychoanalytic emphasis on the past is a retreat from the future and from confrontation with death" (p. 19). The recognition of such denial and the subsequent "awakening" of our psyche to life's finitude can be achieved more often at critical junctures of life such as the loss of a loved one, critical illness, significant milestones of life, change in career, or your relationship status. Yalom's book was written in 2018, so it doesn't explicitly add pandemics to the list but does mention the general category of "cataclysmic trauma," which will obviously include the sudden onset of the Covid-19 pandemic. Yalom illustrates this awakening with several examples, but one of them stands out for its literary and existential insights. He refers to Tolstoy's "The Death of Ivan Ilych," whose eponymous protagonist "shielded himself from the notion of death through his preoccupation with prestige, appearance, and money" only to get overwhelmed by its eventual arrival in the form of a terminal illness into ceaseless screaming for several days before he dies (p. 35). This is a clear instance of what existentialist philosophers would call "anxiety," a state in which one is shaken out of the slumber of everyday existence and forced to confront the meaning of one's life, relationships, values, possibilities, and choices. Death, in other words, forces Ivan Ilych to think about the kind of life he has lived so far, its meaning, fulfillment, and authenticity. He becomes painfully aware of the "nullity" at the heart of existence, of his own being, finitude, and the impossibility of making infinite choices at any stage of life and none after death (Heidegger, 1962, p. 331). With a lot of bitterness and consternation, he realizes that he has probably lived his life the wrong way, but it's too late to make any changes in his career, relationships, or life routines or to make his family members ponder the significance of death because they are too busy with the possibilities and glimmer of life. Eventually, he begins to form loving, compassionate relationships with people who don't deny his impending death (such as his attendant), having understood it as the eventual conclusion of all lives. However, the terror of death overwhelms his final days, and he dies only after screaming ceaselessly for several days.

For the purpose of this chapter, we will examine another literary illustration of denial of death, a denial that manifests as a desire for reckless partying rather than work during the times of the Covid-19 pandemic. The following sections of this chapter will read Udayan Mukherjee's "The Party" (included in *Essential Items and Other Tales from a Land in Lockdown*, 2020), a story about a posh party hosted during the Covid-19 pandemic, as an instance of "play" and extend it to the cultural practice of partying in general. "The Party" is a short story about the experiences of an unnamed narrator (who is often addressed as "Sandy" by others) at a party thrown by his friend Rahul that includes other guests like the businessman Ronnie; his wife Pixy, "author of popular Parsi cookbooks"; Madhav, who "headed an online education start-up"; "Ajay, the hotelier, and his gallerist wife, Madhu." The upper-class composition of the group attending the party suggested by this brief selection of occupations is corroborated by claims made by the narrator's wife about their unnamed housing complex ("if there was a case in this place, the entire AIIMS staff would be in attendance," p. 73); the excitement around the dramatic return of Reema, the host's daughter, from the United States just before "the shutters came down" made possible by a hefty sum of money; the mention of "two drinks trollies, one with the wines and spirits, the other with mixers and ice buckets" (p. 75) at the party made possible by paying the price multiple times the marked price; and helps like Nandu who were designated to tend to these trollies. Before Sandy attends the party, he has a conversation with his wife, Tania, about it, whose immediate response is laughter. "You are joking, right?" she asks, and the narrator finds himself agreeing initially:

> Who could even think of throwing a terrace party at a time like this? Yet, I couldn't deny that I was interested. The prospect of being around people after such a long time, sharing a drink, having a few laughs together—seemed attractive.
>
> *(p. 70)*

While Tania hazards the possibility that her husband wants to go simply because he is "stifled" and "stuck" with her in a "house arrest" precipitated by the lockdown guidelines issued by the state during the early months of the pandemic, the husband avoids any confrontation and decides to go to the party without her. He does admit that the parties thrown by Rahul are often driven by alcohol, capital, and bombast:

> Rahul's gatherings degenerated, as she had described, into piss-ups. And Tania's presence, with her judging eyes and aura of disapproval, acted like a harness, constantly pulling me back from the edge of abandonment. I could always tell she was filing away titbits to bring up later, to prove to me that I wasn't essentially very different from those other braggarts.
>
> *(p. 71)*

Perhaps this is precisely what he needed after several months of being locked in his own house, thinking about disease and death. Toward the end of the evening, he declares: "Madhav's words, about being able to give till it pinched (the reference to donating to the needy), sloshed uneasily in my head, as did the fumes from the parting shot of brandy Rahul had forced on me." That is, alcohol and all that it enables—sociability, tolerance (of some people Rahul clearly doesn't like), and a break from or forgetting of the world outside the party, which included the pandemic and the specter of death it had unleashed—remains the resonant note for all conversations and activities that happen at the party. What, we must ask, is so attractive about alcohol and partying, especially when people around you are dying unpredictably after catching a deadly virus and you have been advised to avoid such gatherings? What, we must ask, is so attractive about "piss-ups," as Rahul puts it?

In *Alcohol: Social Drinking in Cultural Context* (2013), Janet Chrzan provides a possible answer. Her argument is that many adults in contemporary United States (and other countries with similar cultures) "use alcohol as a semiotic sign that signals or frames leisure" (p. 83), especially after the arrival of "industrial time" and a "protestant work ethics" associated with capitalism that produces rigid, regimented lives and schedules, using dichotomies of work/play, sober diligence/drunk carnival, etc., whereby people are expected to adopt different behaviors and identities during workdays/work hours and weekends/parties (p. 86). This was obviously not the case for earlier historical periods when leisure wasn't so sharply divided from work, and people could pursue demanding, meaningful skills even during hours allocated to leisure. Using the analysis of everyday rhythms by Henri Lefebvre, Chrzan points out that alcohol, and the associated space for partying that it enables, act as a cue to shift identities from work-self to play/leisure-self, allowing for a tolerance of behavior that would not be tolerated otherwise (e.g., puking in public, flirting). She argues further that the oscillation between these two poles of the binaries often creates an addiction to both—work-related stress, the sense of being busy and multitasking for success, and the carnivalesque release from such stress in the form of a "time-out" or "piss-ups" where everyone gets "hammered" and "checks out" in a way (p. 93). Chrzan adds:

> Alcohol facilitates this transformation because it is anti-linear time, encourages submersion in the moment, the social group and the event. Time is lost as intoxication and sociality take over. The cultural actor ignores the clock and loses control. The sober worker unbound becomes free, spontaneous and 'authentic'—characteristics released and promoted by alcohol use. Alcohol becomes a symbol and sign of leisure, of free time, authenticity of self and of social life. *(p. 96)*

In short, alcohol, especially within the social setting of a party, activates a domain of play as opposed to the domain of work and everyday reality. This play works, of course, on the individual level as well as collective: the individual, if they believe that one is not their regular self once drunk, can rationalize certain behaviors and statements that they wouldn't be able to explain if they are assumed to be originating from their sober self, thus "get(ting) it out of their systems" with a minimum of adverse consequences" (p. 81).

The domain of play has been theorized variously in philosophy and cultural studies. In "A Pluralist Conception of Play," Randolph Feezell (2013) has helpfully outlined some of these crucial ways of understanding this phenomenon by providing a list of elements that demarcates the "family resemblances" that define play. These elements include freedom (to participate and follow certain rules); autotelicity (or the performance of certain activities for their own sake, without any external motives, as may be the case with most activities that constitute work); some order of make-believe or "un-reality," created, for instance, by inserting unnecessary modifications, obstacles, complexities, and rules (e.g., the rules employed in a game of soccer or cricket); a "suspension of the ordinary"; and a transition to a mode of life/space-time/causality that's different from the ordinary mode of existence, diminishing of the consciousness of self and its absorption into the activity or the collective, activation of new ways of thinking, communicating, operating, moving, and acting, propelled by a "serious nonseriousness," "uncertainty, spontaneity, improvisation—and fun" (p. 23). These attributes help us understand the ways in which the domain of play (be it a party in the pandemic or the Coronavirus challenge) brackets the reality that constitutes its antithesis. Hilde Hein (1968) reiterates Freud's observations about traumatic events that recur in dreams or as part of children's play to make this clearer. Freud links such repetitions to an aggressive attempt on the subject's part (triggered by a death instinct that intends to return the body to the peaceful state of nonexistence) to master or overcome the painful situation they may have undergone or witnessed, thus turning play into active conquest of passive setbacks (p. 69). "Challenging" the virus or the death it signified through the "Coronavirus challenge" would thus seem like a reasonable response to the sudden and unpredictable deaths around us caused by a pandemic that one didn't understand clearly. Heine also underlines the fact that "play provides a means of escaping reality and therein lies its value" while noting that "in a world in which everyone was perfectly adapted to reality there would be no need for either play or art" (p. 69).

One would possibly not need to "get hammered" and "party like an animal" if reality did not have painful experiences like death, hunger, and disappointments. Alternatively, one would probably not feel the need to party in a pandemic if everyone were willing to authentically engage with its reality, considering the meaning and significance of death for life in the pandemic. It must be noted here that play—be it in the form of a viral game, party, or artwork—doesn't always constitute an unphilosophical escape from or a nullification of reality. Sandy, the narrator of Mukherjee's story, repeatedly compares the party to a play, reminding us of the logic of play shared by a party and work of art: "The champagne was going down nicely," he says, "I had the distinct impression of watching a play in which all the actors were personally known to me" (p. 79). When the party's over, he feels that "the play was nearing an end, only the feast remained" (p. 87). Art, which allows us to play with elements of reality within its domain by opening up possibilities and insights unavailable to us in the real world, has its own "seriousness," its singular way of making sense of and shaping reality using certain perspectives, rules, and injunctions (Homan, 2013, p. 100). In an article titled "Whoever Cannot Give, Also Receives Nothing: Nietzsche's Playful Spectator," Catherine Homan reminds us that while we are playing, we always keep the real world in view somehow, draw from it, maintain an oblique relationship with it:

> [W]e remain in a productive tension with what is distant from us, and what is distant from us actually draws us to it. We do not leave it behind but continue to hold it in our sight from another perspective.
> *(p. 102)*

The same paragraph quotes Nietzsche's *The Gay Science*:

> At times we need a rest from ourselves by looking upon, by looking down upon ourselves and, from an artistic distance, laughing over ourselves or weeping over ourselves.... [W]e need all exuberant, floating, dancing, mocking, childish, and blissful art lest we lose the freedom above things that our ideal demands of us.... We should be able to also ... float above it and play.
> *(p. 102)*

This implies, Homan suggests, that should the subject be committed enough, the possibilities, freedom, and creativity gleaned from art can be transferred to reality, turning life into play, so that we respond to the challenges, crises (of meaning or practicalities), and anxieties of life with a spirit of play. While walking back to his house after the party, Sandy witnesses a tender moment in the dark: a couple, a "night guard" and a "live-in maid," sitting together on a bench, "next to the overgrown crepe Jasmine bush." When he sees that the boy is trying to console the crying girl, he decides not to disturb them, leaving us with this rhetorical question as the story ends: "Who knew what private griefs they nursed in their young hearts?" (p. 88). Perhaps the hours spent watching "the play" of the party have awakened Sandy's artistic, aesthetic sensibility, and he finds that the only response to some grief is (the beauty of) silence. The question of whether Sandy would bring back any insights gathered during "play" into life and would take this sensibility further by looking at the possibilities, challenges, and events of life in the pandemic creatively, playfully, and authentically remains unanswered at the end of the story.

To extend the problematic of this paper, I will point out that willful denial or defiance of death of the kind we have been discussing also points to a possible analytical framework for understanding the general manner in which the pandemic was experienced by many of us, irrespective of whether we chose to play, philosophize or perish. To most people, the early days of the pandemic were deeply shocking and unsettling, generating anxiety-centered moods that later stabilized into chronic anxiety, sadness, or anger. Some of these attributes characterize moods associated with what Sigmund Freud famously analyzed as "the uncanny" (2003). In his essay, Freud explores the etymologies and semantic fields of the terms *heimlich* (canny/homely) and *unheimlich* (uncanny/unhomely) to emphasize their overlap instead of distinction. Freud highlights the dialectic of these two terms by pointing out the linkage between what is homely/familiar and what is unhomely/familiar/secretive/concealed: what is homely must appear unhomely to the outsider. At the same time, a secondary meaning of *unheimlich* is that which has been uncovered or revealed. This brings us to the curious linkage between the meanings of the two words and a possible definition of the uncanny: Freud defines it as "the species of the frightening that goes back to what was once well known and had long been familiar," that is, the "return" of what was "repressed" and, therefore, once familiar (say, castration complex or primary narcissism that are usually suppressed or repressed on the route to adulthood). If Yalom is correct about the force of death anxiety in our lives, it is a repressed component that's bound to return as the uncanny. This could explain the shock, awe, and bewilderment that characterized the early days of the pandemic (e.g., the response of people everywhere as they learned how to carry on their lives with masks on, to stay inside because death lurked outside and to make sense of empty roads as well as the high toll of Covid-19 patients in countries like the United States and India) as if people were suddenly reminded of the fact that their loved ones and their own selves were mortal and death was an unavoidable, unpredictable eventuality for the human individual as well as the species.

A lot of this anger, of course, turned into outright denial of the damage that the virus could cause as well as the death toll (Funke and Sanders, 2020). Regimes, leaders, and people across the world had heated debates about whether Covid-19 is more dangerous than the common cold or simply a "hoax," and whether Coronavirus could kill you at all if you didn't have any comorbidities (which it totally could back then), and whether wearing masks did anything at all to protect the user or ended up damaging the health of the wearer. An article on Kaiser Health News' website tells us that conspiracy theories popped up everywhere, making bizarre claims like "a 26-minute video called "Plandemic: The Hidden Agenda Behind Covid-19" (2021), wherein a former scientist at the National Cancer Institute claimed the virus was manipulated in a lab, hydroxychloroquine is effective against coronaviruses, and face masks make people sick." By way of another example, KHN tells us:

> ...Fox News featured a guest who opened a new misinformation assault on hospitals.
>
> Dr. Scott Jensen, a Minnesota physician, and Republican state senator, told Ingraham that, because hospitals were receiving more money for Covid-19 patients on Medicare—a result of a coronavirus stimulus bill—they were overcounting Covid-19 cases. He had no proof of fraud, but the cynical story took off.
>
> *(Funke and Sanders, 2020)*

The characters in Mukherjee's story have an elaborate debate about whether partying or playing loud music would be okay if everybody around them was a little "jumpy," and whether the government should lift the lockdown restrictions simply because it was causing boredom and economic distress among the rich (with lip service to the cause of the daily worker—*presswallahs*, vegetable vendors, auto drivers—a claim whose hypocrisy is quickly pointed out when Madhav proposes a combined donation effort and most of the guests refuse to contribute anything substantial while talking about buying expensive stocks, paintings, and wine in the same breath) and whether the government should impose additional taxes on the rich. When the conversation gets a tad serious and heated, everybody agrees to go back to talking about stocks and paintings, as if the situation caused by the pandemic did not warrant the time and seriousness that conversation was about to extract.

Such denial is the opposite of what existentialist philosophers call "authenticity," that is, analyzing the brute reality, painful aspects, and meaninglessness of our lives (and deaths) in order to live a life in accordance with the values of our choice. This can only be achieved by what Heidegger (1962) called "being-towards-death," that is, facing up to and embracing one's finitude and mortality instead of denying it through work or play (p. 293). Only such an approach to life can restore to each choice the weight and significance accorded by our finitude: one can only choose so many times and pursue so many projects before one faces death which, to quote Heidegger again, is the "impossibility" of possibilities. Doing this will generate anxiety, of course, in the conventional as well as existential sense. However, the existentialist philosophers valued anxiety instead of fearing it because it pointed to the lack of any absolute meanings in our lives (given to us by God, state, family, etc.) and, therefore, to the exhilarating but terrifying freedom of creating meaning through our decisions, actions, and values. This anxiety, however, unlike the fear that we are familiar with, doesn't have any specific cause/object to attach itself but the very fact of our existence, our life and death, and is, therefore, more unsettling and terrifying. The Covid-19 pandemic certainly triggered such anxiety for many of us. Our response, like the guests at the party in Mukherjee's story, was varied. While some of us partied and played together, some of us perished, "each alone" (Cowper, 1799), giving in to the anxiety and letting it manifest as a symptom, a constant presence, or an existential awakening. Like the group "Guilty Remnant" in the HBO TV series *Leftovers*, who constantly remind people of their loved ones who disappeared mysteriously one fine day by wearing white and smoking incessantly, without ever saying a word, some of us took this to the other extreme of partying by repeatedly reminding people of the possibility of death that the pandemic was a synecdoche for, reminding them that in the end, death comes for us all, those who deny it and those who learn the art of living from it:

> No voice divine the storm allay'd,
> No light propitious shone;
> When, snatch'd from all effectual aid,
> We perish'd, each alone:
> But I beneath a rougher sea,
> And whelm'd in deeper gulfs than he.
>
> (Cowper, 1799)

A few of us learned how to play in a committed, mindful way so that we did not perish at the hands of life, staring at the sun of life/death but blinking at it flirtatiously.

References

Chrzan, J. (2013) *Alcohol: Social Drinking in Cultural Context*. New York: Routledge.

Cowper, W. (1799) The Castaway. [online] Poetry Foundation. Available at: https://www.poetryfoundation.org/poems/44027/the-castaway

Feezell, R. (2013) A Pluralist Conception of Play. In: E. Ryall, E.W. Russell, and M. MacLean (eds.) *The Philosophy of Play* (pp. 11–31). New York: Routledge.

Freud, S. (2003) *The Uncanny*. London: Penguin.

Funke, D. and Sanders, K. (2020) Lie of the Year: The Downplay and Denial of the Coronavirus. [online] *KFF Health News*. Available at: https://kffhealthnews.org/news/article/lie-of-the-year-the-downplay-and-denial-of-thecoronavirus/ (Accessed 8 July, 2024).

Heidegger, M. (1962) *Being and Time*. Oxford: Blackwell Publishers.

Hein, H. (1968) Play as an Aesthetic Concept. *The Journal of Aesthetics and Art Criticism*, 27(1), 67–71.

Homan, C. (2013) Whoever Cannot Give, Also Receives Nothing: Nietzsche's Playful Spectator. In: E. Ryall, E.W. Russell, and M. MacLean (eds.) *The Philosophy of Play* (pp. 98–108). New York: Routledge.

Kamphorst, J. (2008) *In Praise of Death: History and Poetry in Medieval Marwar (South Asia)*. Leiden: Leiden University Press.

Mukherjee, U. (2020) *Essential Items and Other Tales from a Land in Lockdown*. New Delhi: Bloomsbury.

The Times of India. (2020) Coronavirus Challenge on TikTok: Video Maker Infected After Licking Public Toilet Seat. [online] Available at: https://timesofindia.indiatimes.com/gadgets-news/coronavirus-challenge-on-tiktok-video-maker-infected-after-licking-public-toilet-seat/articleshow/74839613.cms# (Accessed 3 July, 2024).

Yalom, I.D. (2008) *Staring at the Sun: Overcoming the Terror of Death*. San Francisco: Jossey-Bass.

PART 3

Pandemic Transitions

From Physical to Virtual

7

TEACHING (IN) PANDEMIC

Lessons Lost, Lessons Learned

James S. Baumlin

What follows is a meditation on the effects—personal and institutional—that Covid-19 has had on classroom instruction. The classroom here described belongs to creative nonfiction (a.k.a. "the personal essay"), a college-level writing course in which the lived experience of students provides much of the subject matter.[1] By its writing assignments and in-class discussions, such a course serves to unmask the several social, economic, environmental, and health crises affecting students today. These, demonstrably, have raised students' levels of anxiety and depression, heightening their feelings of isolation and lack of direction, driving some to panic, some to despair, and some (by no means all) to a benumbing indifference. It's easy to name these as so many symptoms of this-or-that condition, but what American popular culture has left unspoken (and, hence, hidden from students) are the external material/ideological *causes* of their distress. We treat anxiety/depression as so much "private property" belonging to the individual, whereas its causes are collective and precede Covid-19.

While the pandemic proved costly to teaching—hence, the "Lessons Lost" figured in this present essay's title—it has also highlighted struggles (intellectual, affective, existential) that students were already experiencing prior to the pandemic but hadn't yet named or confronted directly. In effect, the pandemic "made visible" aspects of American popular culture that needed to be called out and critiqued. Incorporated into our living classroom discussion, these are the "Lessons Learned," again as referenced in the title.

The concern of this present essay reaches beyond teaching to the problem of personal knowledge per se: hence the epigraph from Michael Polanyi, whose epistemology of "tacit knowing" treats knowledge as a

DOI: 10.4324/9781003590392-11

crisis, not just of certitude but of communication. In the well-worn Polanyian formula, "we believe more than we can prove and know more than we can say" (Nixon, 2012, p. 58). Polanyi thus provides the starting point for a critique of American popular culture—which, as Slavoj Žižek suggests, imposes its "will-to-ignorance" (or, more forcefully, the "will not-to-know") on Covid-19 and its impact on health, community/sociality, politics, and economy.[2] To say that we dwell in a post-fact, post-truth age reinforces Žižek's point. In invoking Polanyi as a counter to this willed ignorance, one returns to distinctions made many decades ago in his *Personal Knowledge*.

There are a number of assumptions, each interrelated, lurking in this present essay; these are listed briefly below.

1 All-knowing is personal. Such is a thesis of Michael Polanyi's influential book, which sought to conjoin "facts" (traditionally the "stuff' of sciences) to "values" (traditionally the province of the humanities). More than a half-century later, we remain engaged in this fact/value debate. Intellectually, we may follow Polanyi in bridge-building across disciplines, but the distinctions between these terms abide: defining our ways of being-in-the-world, these mark our equal commitments to "what is" (i.e., to the world of facts) and "what ought to be" (i.e., to a stable, shared firmament of values).
2 To that first claim, it can be added that all *writing* is "personal." For writing, being one of intellectual culture's privileged "ways of knowing," reflects an author's commitments, aspirations, and complex humanity. It's upon this humane basis that we can ground an ethic of discourse: we expect authors "to stand behind their words" or, put baldly, *to mean what they say* (or write). Such an ethic treats all writing, when value-laden, as an implicit "personal essay." The idealistic assumption here is that we speak or write in good faith, responsible for our own words while remaining open—responsive—to the words of others.
3 To this ethical idealism, one can add a more boldly existentialist claim: specifically, that our works are *embodiments* of the words that belong to the voice that speaks them or the hand that writes them, in each case translating thought into bodily gesture. We say that authors "stand behind their words" when speaking or writing in good faith; within an incarnational rhetoric, we might say that authors stand *in* their words, energizing them, filling them with passionate commitment and intention. It's by our embodiments that we make knowledge "personal," wedding fact-claims to values in "a perpetual incarnation" (Bozarth-Campbell, 1979, p. 116).[3]

4 When pursued as a "way of knowing," all writing is personal. By analogy, it can be argued that all *teaching*—concomitantly, all *learning*—is personal. In any classroom setting, facts "belong" to the external/material subject or discipline, to which teachers attach specific personal commitments and, by embodying these, serve to put them "on display." To profess a discipline requires more than a dispassionate command of terms and concepts; rather, the professor's "way of knowing" becomes gestural—a "way of being-in-the-world," *of embodying and performing* the work of one's discipline. The very vocation of teaching-as-professing celebrates the Polanyian wedding of fact and value, consciousness and corporeity. Teacherly "personal knowing" seeks its witness and fulfillment in student-responsiveness: that is, in the student's own reciprocal actions of learning.[4] Ideally, teaching translates into "studenting," its mirror double.

5 As Polanyi describes it, "personal knowing" stands opposed to an ideology of individualism, "rugged" or otherwise, such as it dominates in the United States today. It is, rather, an epistemology tied to an ethic of responsible discourse, one that conjoins material facts to humane values while opening its claims to public scrutiny and response. Trained as a chemist, Polanyi intended his theory to serve as a hedge against individualist bias in science. Giving up assumptions of objectivity and impersonality, science describes *a model of communication* whose practitioners aim to serve the wider community; they do so by "policing" their discourse, and remaining open to testing and public debate. In our own politically divided post-fact, science-skeptic, pandemic-torn world, we remain in desperate need of the Polanyian model.

Such are the premises underlying paragraphs that follow.

Lessons Lost

During the height of the Covid-19 pandemic, classroom teaching had been replaced by online instruction, much of it scripted and videotaped. Needless to say, this retreat from the classroom entailed a loss. Previously, throughout a 40-year career in teaching, the author of this present essay had experienced the classroom as a living, dynamic, and surprising swirl. More than an exchange of information, classroom teaching had come to describe an exchange *of energy*. (And how could it be otherwise, when living breathing passionate embodied human beings are engaged?) While some readers might find this puzzling or surprising, it's in the full confidence of personal experience that this claim is being made.[5]

Put simply, there's more to teaching than an exchange of information.

To illustrate, here's the story of a teacher who learned this lesson the hard way, through online coursework in Shakespeare.[6] For this teacher, the basic facts of the bard's life and writings were well known and easily strung together, as in the following imaginary video-lecture:

> Born in 1564 to Stratford glover John Shakespeare, William married Ann Hathaway in 1582 when he was 18 and she 26 (and several months pregnant). He wrote his earliest of 39 known plays by 1591, *Hamlet* in 1600, *King Lear* in 1606, *The Tempest* in 1610. He died in 1616 at age 54. Compiled by fellow players John Heminges and Henry Condell, the First Folio of his plays appeared in 1623. *What else do you want to know?*

What else, indeed. The reader might ask, "How is 'mere' information of this sort the stuff of teaching? Here are 'facts' aplenty, but where are the 'values' to wed them? Where, indeed, is their human face?" Nothing in the facts themselves express that committed, passionate, *personal* knowledge so prized by Polanyi; surely the dates, names, and titles inform teaching, but they remain "dead letters" in themselves.

Having spent two years of classroom-banished instruction making PowerPoint slideshows and videotaping lectures on Shakespeare's life, times, and writings, the teacher found himself suddenly *addicted to information*. Though returned to the living breathing classroom, he felt an urge, indeed an urgency, to replicate all the information that he had gathered, scripted, and recorded for consumption online. In effect, the teacher had turned himself into a delivery system. Prior to the pandemic, his classroom teaching had been governed by personal insights and intuition: the teacher would walk into the room, wait for the words to come, and find the persons who most needed to hear them. Questions were asked and answered, leading to further questioning and answering.

It has taken more than a year for this teacher to remember how the *living* classroom felt—and *how the teacher himself felt* in that living, swirling classroom. It's a place of teaching and learning, of course, but it comes alive when treated as a place *of experiencing* teaching and learning. Sometimes, we need to remind ourselves of the existential nature of face-to-face instruction, something that the pandemic took from us, if temporarily.

At its best, classroom teaching describes an *event* wherein something surprising, something *unscripted*, can occur by virtue of the fact that two or more people face each other within a safe shared space, mindful of each other's needs and interests and willing to take risks in their sharing. Teaching seeks "to open a space" between people, a space where minds can meet and cohabit. Language opens that space, but more than language is involved: the risk-taking inscribed in teaching entails a language of passionate personal commitment wedded to bodily gestures. The teacher's classroom presence is, as Polanyi implies, a bodily presence. Much as one's words, one's body overflows with expressive meaning, and it's bodily presence that makes classroom teaching preeminently ethical.[7] Our capacity to stand ethically within this shared linguistic space rests in our human capacity for response.

Mikhail Bakhtin ascribes a similar function to art. For the great Russian theorist, all genuine art (i.e., art unsullied by propaganda) is marked by "answerability" (Bakhtin, 1990, p. 2). Such is the humane value of art generally and of writing specifically: our works invite questions, which in turn seek out answers, their ultimate destination being an answer word. Note that answerability is the opposite of authority: any questions posed by propaganda reduce to mere catechism—to a rehearsing of the already-assumed, which demands our obedience to the already-spoken and deafness to the as-yet unspoken. Authentic questions address real-world problems without placing limits or preconditions upon one's answering. And no question is worth asking if the answer is already known and settled. Often we err in declaring a problem "solved." In life as in teaching, the problems that we confront are generative. They are never fully, finally, and forever answered, *but they are answerable.*[8] In the epigraph cited above, Polanyi declares the "inherently hazardous" nature of intellectual commitments; the hazard of one's "personal knowing" rests in its open public display, for which the author remains personally, and ethically responsible.

Answerability belongs to the classroom, as well. Teaching properly so-called occurs when teacher and student, each engaged in questioning and answering, trade places. For that's when students discover and declare their own passionate commitments—their own personal knowing—in ways surprising to all engaged. This surprising, unscripted moment may be rare; not all students in all classrooms experience it. But it does happen. It's the opposite of catechism, and it's what students and teachers live for.

Here, then, is what the teacher lost during our pandemic-driven retreat from the classroom: the freedom to throw away scripted instruction, in order to experience the living breathing classroom both *as an exchange of energy* within a shared linguistic space and *as a structure of surprise* inspiring new ways of speaking and knowing, forever open to questioning, infinitely answerable.

And what of our students? What did they lose, particularly in the early months of the pandemic when classrooms were closed and social distancing imposed?

It's in the experience of our students that we discover the fragility of our shared public spaces, particularly when discourse moves from the classroom to the wilderness of media-driven pop culture. In the open form of popular discourse, language is too often desecrated and disabled, shorn of its epistemic powers. When viewed critically from the political left-of-center, one sees an America whose political-economic institutions wield power *by the destruction of discourse as a shared, responsive, answerable intellectual space.* As Marker Fisher writes, "Contemporary culture has eliminated both the concept of the public and the figure of the intellectual. Former public spaces—both physical and cultural—are now either derelict or colonized by advertising. A cretinous anti-intellectualism presides" (Fisher, 2009, p. 82). And a primary effect of this anti-intellectualism is a willed ignorance regarding the causes of our societal ills. This ignorance, as Žižek puts it, is the "will not-to-know."

To elaborate: what some party politics, some institutions of government, some modes of education, some media outlets, and some practitioners of science, technology, and even healthcare impose is a willed ignorance *that fails to question* the "facts" claimed and "values" asserted in popular discourse. Žižek writes of this failure in *PANDEMIC! 2: Chronicles of a Time Lost*, and its effect can be charted in students' work. As noted above, the author of this present essay regularly teaches coursework in creative nonfiction, sections of which were offered online, in the midst of the Covid-19 storm. In these sections, students were asked to write about their experiences. Several themes recurred. These included a prevailing sense of loneliness made worse by self-isolation at home; a weakened sense of social identity (often ascribed to the wearing of masks); a quieting of speech (with telegraphic texting as a "conversational" replacement); a sensation of drifting, of living passively without plan or purpose; a retreat from the so-called "real world" into virtual reality (through social media avatars and video-gaming); and, underlying it all, a hefty increase in anxiety and depression. Most of these conditions were not caused by Covid-19, though the pandemic heightened students' feelings of isolation and depression; rather, Covid-19 made these conditions visible. In so doing, the pandemic loosened the veil of ignorance regarding the causes of our collective distress.

Lessons Learned

It's not the virus alone that has killed more than a million citizens of the United States. Striking at a time of extreme partisan politics, Covid-19 has had help. Even as the nation overcame its initial shock and worked to develop protocols—social distancing, masking, the closing of restaurants and other public spaces—Americans began dying *of ideology*. Science-skepticism, mistrust of "big government," and the conviction that public health policies violated individual freedom: such attitudes circulated throughout the nation's conservative electorate, effectively doubling its death rate.[9] Historically, Americans have laid aside differences to band together, either for a common purpose or against a common enemy. Had we agreed "to declare war" against Covid-19, many thousands of lives would have been spared; instead, a large portion of the electorate "declared war" against communitarian policies, choosing "individual freedoms" over public health.

And yet, for all its waste and suffering, the pandemic may bring some good after all. It may do so by pulling the veil from the American ideology and its dream of unfettered freedom—an ideology wherein individuals solely are responsible for their own happiness and where any failure in the pursuit of that happiness belongs to the individual and not to the institutions, constraints, and control mechanisms of culture. To quote from Fisher:

> The "methodological individualism" of the capitalist realist worldview ... regards notions such as the public as "spooks," phantom abstractions devoid of content. *All that is real is the individual (and their families)*. The symptoms of the failures of this worldview are everywhere—in a disintegrated social sphere in which teenagers shooting each other has become commonplace, in which hospitals incubate aggressive superbugs—what is required is that effect be connected to structural causes. Against the postmodernist suspicion of grand narratives, we need to reassert that, far from being isolated, contingent problems, these are all the effects of a single systemic cause: Capital.
>
> *(2009, p. 77; emphasis added)*

As Fisher deploys the term, "capitalist realism" treats free-market capitalism as the new global ontology, totalizing and ineluctable. It's been said that it's easier to imagine the end of the world than to imagine the end of capitalism. In the United States, yes. As Žižek (2020) notes, "the freedom we have in the liberal anarchy of commerce is the freedom to act egotistically (determined by our nature) in a world of exchange that appears as an objective order on which we depend" (pp. 123–124). "What is needed," Žižek (2020) adds, "is a re-politicization of the economy: economic life should be controlled and regulated by the free decisions of a community, not left to the blind, chaotic interaction of market forces" (p. 124). He's right in calling for some version of democratic socialism (for the nonce, let's call it "capitalism with a conscience"). But while this system thrives in some nations (particularly in the Global North), the very term "socialism" has been demonized by American right-wing politics.

By the time this present essay is published, the author's students in creative nonfiction will have finished up their senior-year writing projects and graduated; and, in the meantime, American politics will have continued its rightward drift into neoconservatism. The "will not-to-know" was already strong in these students, who began the course with little to no knowledge of the distinctions among democratic socialism, neoliberalism, and neoconservatism. This ignorance is unsettling, though unsurprising. In response to their personal essays, their teacher-led discussion on these topics, which most (not all) of his students initially thought strange: *Why mention politics in a writing class, for goodness' sake?* Quite effectively, in fact, their education had prepared them for their future lives and careers: they *will* work and they *will* consume, fiercely obedient to the "will not-to-know."

Or, by the self-reflection afforded in writing, they will learn to make their life and work conditions *visible*. Naming these would be the first step in developing personal knowledge that would allow them to rise above their current conditions and stand in a position of critique. And the most pressing task facing these students is a cultural critique of their own "medicalized depression."

Against the "Will Not-to-Know": Writing and Teaching Otherwise

In the state of Missouri where the author currently teaches, one of the most common medical diagnoses (which is typically treated pharmacologically) is anxiety and its mirror-twin, depression. Facts and stats back up this claim. Depression is rampant among college-age students; so much so, that it constitutes an epidemic in itself.[10] In medicalizing depression, we treat it as private property—as something that arises from within and belongs to the individual, whereas the causes of depression (among other expressions of emotional distress) are environmental, economic, political, social, and interpersonal.

The "will not-to-know" comes once again into play, since few if any physicians will talk to their patients about the underlying socioeconomic conditions that fuel their distress. It's effectively taboo: the institutions aimed at safeguarding health will never tell our students the true full cause of their unhappiness—which, as it burgeons, turns into depression full-blown. Unhappiness is a prelude to depression, and the United States as it is aplenty. As the title of an *NBC News* web article declares, "Americans are the unhappiest they've been in 50 years." The article begins:

> 2020 has been rough on the American psyche. Folks in the U.S. are more unhappy today than they've been in nearly 50 years.
>
> This bold—yet unsurprising—conclusion comes from the COVID Response Tracking Study, conducted by NORC at the University of Chicago. It finds that just 14% of American adults say they're very happy, down from 31% who said the same in 2018. That year, 23% said they'd often or sometimes felt isolated in recent weeks. Now, 50% say that.
>
> The survey, conducted in late May, draws on nearly a half-century of research from the General Social Survey, which has collected data on American attitudes and behaviors at least every other year since 1972. No less than 29% of Americans have ever called themselves very happy in that survey.

The article cites one Jonathan Berney of Austin, Texas, who said

> that the pandemic—and his resulting layoff as a digital marketing manager for a law firm—caused him to reevaluate everything in his life. While he admits that he's not exactly happy now, that's led to another uncomfortable question: Was he truly happy before the pandemic?

That's a question, indeed, that Covid-19 inspires us to ask. Is it easier to say "I'm depressed" than "I'm unhappy"? Surely the "will not-to-know" is implicated, in that the American ideology equates career success and consumerism with happiness. To think otherwise is un-American. As Fisher (2009) notes, "we must convert widespread mental health problems from medicalized conditions into effective antagonisms. Affective disorders are forms of captured discontent; this disaffection can and must be channeled outwards, directed towards its real cause, Capital" (p. 80).

Fisher's assessment is spot-on, and we have reason to hope that today's college graduates, members of Generation Z, will learn to channel their energies—their aspirations along with their "disaffection" and "captured discontent"—toward real social-economic change. In Covid-19's aftermath, they've had time to rethink their attitudes toward careerism, consumerism, education, the environment, public health, and lifestyle generally. Boldly put, the pandemic changed many of the ways students see and experience the world. Knowing better, they cannot go back. The future that these students face will include economic uncertainties and career stresses and dissatisfactions. But their collective response can bring change to the workplace and marketplace, making these fairer, more accommodating, more inclusive, and more humane; in many places both nationally and globally, these changes are already occurring in the "where" and the "how" and the "with whom" and the "how long" and the "how much" of one's labor and consumption. Pursuing capitalism with a conscience: such, arguably, is the grand enterprise facing Gen Z.

In the above paragraph, it's students whose writing provided the insights, *teaching their teacher what to write*. When the Covid-19 storm first struck, most of them were high school seniors or college freshmen; in effect, they've spent their college years sheltering from its virulence. While further outbreaks are predicted, the major onslaught has passed, in the United States at least. We are back in the classroom. And, compared to online classes taught in 2020–2022, when classrooms closed and social distancing was enforced, their writing has evolved in its response to the pandemic. Though life experiences remain their subject, they are not dwelling on themes of loss or victimhood. Increasingly heroic in spirit, their narratives tell of survival in the present and hope for the future. Many, to their credit, focus on that first major step in their own self-care, which was the decision to seek professional counseling. They earn our praise for having made that decision and for having the courage to write of it.

As has been noted, teaching properly so-called occurs when teacher and student trade places. Touching on the pandemic and depression, on lifestyle and life aspirations, and on careerism among other topics, students' most recent essays have proved surprisingly unscripted and forward-looking. Their writing surprises by its resourcefulness in meeting life challenges, turning personal experience into an artful, engaging, insightful narrative. Their stories speak of a resilience in adversity beyond anything that their teacher may have experienced personally. Their honesty in self-exploration leaves the reader humbled. Their fearlessness in declaring their own passionate commitments—their own personal knowing—shows a capacity for risk-taking that one cannot help but admire. In their rich, complex lifeworld (let's call it the world of Gen Z), their teachers become their students. And that's how it should be. The boundaries of their lifeworld and that of their teachers only partially overlap. (An example: for Gen Z students, self-image and self-worth are no longer defined by labor. For the so-called Baby-Boomers of the mid-20th century, self-worth and work have been equivalent terms.) Our best teacherly task is to join them in exploring *their* world on *their* terms. And the talents that best serve them are our attentiveness, openness, and trust.

In the field of English studies generally, teachers have a further duty to the following. We must remind students that they're political animals and that the "will not-to-know" weighs heavily upon popular culture. At the same time, we need to remind ourselves that the pandemic hit their generation far harder than it did our own—not in terms of hospitalization or morbidity, but in terms of worldview and self-image. (In their "equipment for living," our students, many still in their teens, were works-in-progress, whereas their teachers met the pandemic fully formed. The Boomers and other, older cohorts were knocked down by Covid-19; in contrast, Gen Z was torn apart and remade by it.) It would be folly on anyone's part to presume that "my pandemic" mirrors "their pandemic." Hence, the students must teach the teachers what they've learned.

If we are to join our students in a common writerly purpose, let it be to make health and community our abiding themes. Together, we can embrace writing as an intellectually courageous will-to-know. We'll be answerable to our texts, putting our passionate commitments "on display." We'll stand by our words; indeed, we'll stand *in* them, embodying them. We'll reserve the right to question, even as we stand ready to give an answer. We'll face the facts, however harsh, that the world throws at us. We'll learn to care for ourselves and for each other in mind, body, and spirit. And we'll learn, as we write, to distinguish authentic personal values from externally imposed ideology. These are worthy aspirations, each arising out of and responsive to our experience of pandemic.

Notes

1 Let me declare up front that I write as a teacher in a public university in the American Middle West whose students are blue collar for the most part, with many—a majority, actually—working to put food on the table. While diverse in some other respects (ethnicity, gender, sexual identity), they share insight into their post-graduation futures, having tasted the life of wage labor. It's a senior-level "capstone" course that I'm describing, a "Seminar in English Studies/Public Affairs." Treating writing as a mode of civic engagement, assignments

typically begin in personal narrative and end in cultural critique. (As a model, the present essay reflects this same socially engaged movement through narrative to criticism.).

2 While revising this piece for publication, I toyed with the alternative title, "On the 'Will Not-to-Know'" (or, for a more deconstructive version, "Against the 'Will Not-to-Know': Writing and Teaching Otherwise"). It's too soon to explore this Žižek-inspired term, but I toyed with it for having named a target and topic of my recent teaching.

3 Didn't Covid-19 turn attention to these precious frail living bodies? It may surprise that an essay on pedagogy would focus so strongly on bodily presence and gesture. But in the closing of classrooms and other public spaces, it was our *bodies* that suffered banishment. Indeed, we work and play, we suffer and endure, we experience the world and know ourselves through/in/as bodies. As a point of philosophy, this essay seeks to reassert the body's energetic presence and role in teaching and learning.

For Polanyi, all human instrumentations (linguistic, logical, mathematical) and the "pre-suppositions" that these generate *look to the body as to their habitus*. He writes, "[W]hen we accept a certain set of pre-suppositions and use them as our interpretative framework, we may be said to dwell in them as we do in our own body" (60). Here, Polanyi follows Maurice Merleau-Ponty's nondualistic claims concerning the corporeity of consciousness and intentionality of the body: "Insofar as I have hands, feet, a body, I sustain around me intentions which are not dependent on my decisions and which affect my surroundings in a way that I do not choose" (Merleau-Ponty 440; for further philosophical discussion, see Levinas).

4 I'm equating teaching with learning here, since my definition of the former rests in a demonstration or performance *of how one learns* within one's discipline. (This essay, for example, marks my own classroom contribution on the topic, "writing in an age of pandemic." Intended as a model for their own final project, it was written with, and for, my students in creative nonfiction.).

5 While some readers might treat this energy-exchange as "mere" metaphor, I intend it literally. As a certified practitioner of the Myers-Briggs Type Inventory (MBTI), I'm sensitive to the distinctions between extraverted and introverted teaching/learning styles. Among other typical features, these are marked by the direction in which individuals focus their mental/corporeal energy, with an extravert's directed largely outward—out into the world, as it were—while an introvert's turns largely inward. My own teaching, which is strongly extraverted (and intuitive, to invoke another MBTI dimension), has occasionally exhausted introverted students even as it has energized extraverts. I make this point, because there are indeed some students whose learning styles thrive in the calmer, "cooler shades" of online instruction. (For MBTI applications to teaching and writing, see Jensen and DiTiberio.).

I'm also trained as a practitioner of Reiki. Here, too, some readers will raise doubt. But the modalities of energy medicine—predominantly Eastern in their cultural development and practice—have at last made their way into Western "integrative practice." Witness the following basic text, taken from the website of the renowned Cleveland Clinic:

> Reiki is an energy healing technique that promotes relaxation, reduces stress and anxiety through gentle touch. Reiki practitioners use their hands to deliver energy to your body, improving the flow and balance of your energy to support healing.
>
> Mikao Usui developed reiki in the early 1900s, deriving the term from the Japanese words *rei*, meaning "universal," and *ki*, which refers to the vital life force energy that flows through all living things. Now, reiki is used all over the world, including in hospitals and hospices, to complement other forms of health treatments.
>
> Reiki aids in healing by helping people become energetically balanced—physically, emotionally, mentally and spiritually[.].
>
> ("What Is Reiki?")

I mention these practices (there are others) as widely accepted models of energy manifestation, gathering, and "exchange.".

6 It should not surprise readers to learn that it's the author's own teaching story that's being told.

7 On this incarnational aspect of pedagogy, I'm indebted to theologian Alla Bozarth-Campbell:

> The body converts elements of a situation through its total gesture in response to it. Movement toward another is movement in and of the body, changing the situation by a true inclination. When the body opens itself to others, it finds its own voice in an active coexistence beyond itself. Intention toward another transforms one's bodily existence, which is itself a perpetual incarnation.
>
> (116)

8 Returning to Shakespeare, the great plays continue to generate new meanings suited to each generation; they do so by the openness of the questions asked and the problems posed. Any reading of Shakespeare yields a knowledge that can never be more—nor can it be less—than personal, even when persuasive and spoken on behalf of a community. Being personal, they remain answerable.

9 "Almost twice as many Republicans than Democrats died of Covid," notes Graig Graziosi in the 17 November issue of *The Independent*. Citing a 2021 study published by the National Bureau of Economic Research, Graziosi writes,

> Despite the fact that the initial runs of Covid-19 vaccines were developed during Donald Trump's administration, many

> Republicans and conservatives refused innoculation. Response to the coronavirus pandemic was politicised, resulting in many Republicans refusing to take the vaccine, either as a result of misinformation spread by conspiracy communities and right-wing media figures and lawmakers, or simply due to a lack of trust in the Biden administration.

In an age of pandemic, one's politics can prove deadly.

10 Measuring incidents of depression nationwide, the web article, "Depression in the U.S. – Statistics & Facts" reads as follows:

> The most common age at which adults experienced a major depressive episode as of 2021 was between 18 and 25 years, with up to 27 percent of women aged 18 to 20 years reporting such an episode in the past year. Depression is also common among youth, with up to 29 percent of teenage girls and almost 12 percent of boys experiencing a major depressive episode in the past year as of 2021.

Also reporting in 2021, America's Health Rankings focuses specifically on Missouri's adult population: The "percentage of adults who reported ever being told by a health professional that they have a depressive disorder, including depression, major depression, minor depression or dysthymia" reaches 22.8% ("Depression in Missouri"). Note that these figures treat depression separately from anxiety. Also, needless to say, they do not account for incidences that go undiagnosed and unreported.

Bibliography

Bakhtin, M.M. (1990) Art and Answerability. In: M. Holquist and V. Liapnov (eds.) *Art and Answerability: Early Philosophical Essays*. Translated by V. Liapunov. Texas: Texas University Press, pp. 1–3.

Bozarth-Campbell, A. (1979) *The Word's Body: An Incarnational Aesthetic of Interpretation*. Alabama: University of Alabama Press.

Cleveland Clinic. (2021) What Is Reiki? [online] Available at: https://health.clevelandclinic.org/reiki/ (Accessed 20 April 2023).

Fisher, M. (2009) *Capitalist Realism: Is There No Alternative?* London: Zero Books.

Jensen, G.H. and DiTiberio, J.K. (1995) *Writing and Personality*. Boston: Davies-Black.

Levinas, E. (1969) *Totality and Infinity: An Essay on Exteriority*. Translated by A. Lingis. Pennsylvania: Duquesne University Press.

Merleau-Ponty, M. (2012) *Phenomenology of Perception*. Translated by D.A. Landes. London and New York: Routledge.epw.

NBC News. (2020) Americans are the Unhappiest They've Been in 50 Years, Poll Finds. [online] Available at: https://www.nbcnews.com/politics/politics-news/americans-are-unhappiest-they-ve-been50-years-poll-finds-n1231153 (Accessed 25 May 2023).

Nixon, J. (2012) *Interpretive Pedagogies for Higher Education: Arendt, Berger, Said, Nussbaum and Their Legacies*. New York: Continuum.
Polanyi, M. (2012) *Personal Knowledge: Towards a Post-Critical Philosophy*. Chicago: University of Chicago Press.
Statista. (2023) Depression in the U.S. – Statistics & Facts. [online] Available at: https://www.statista.com/topics/4569/depression-in-the-us/#topicOverview (Accessed 25 May 2023).
United Health Foundation. (2023) Depression in Missouri. [online] Available at: https://www.americashealthrankings.org/explore/measures/Depression_a/MO (Accessed 25 May 2023).
Žižek, S. (2020) *PANDEMIC! 2: Chronicles of a Time Lost*. New York: Polity Press.

8

CYBER IN THE PANDEMIC ART

Armeen Kaur Ahuja

Art is probably the most sacred form of intimacy. But is intimacy strictly human? Or can it exist beyond the human? And most importantly, beyond the organic? Quarantine protocols pushed the human species to the edge of their sensory spectrum. The long tradition of creating and perceiving art had been dependent on inspiration born of an ecosystem that was, if not organic, at least naturalized. The lockdown in the pandemic came as an axe upon this lineage of tradition. The world surrounding artists suddenly went bleak, the tradition of seeing, feeling, and getting inspired required a revival; a house was no longer a home but an enclosure, thereby upturning the narratives of *comfort* and *discomfort*. Artists now required a window to look outside the enclosure, but even if they found the window, it did not come with a view.

This attempt to look beyond the enclosure that turned the digital world into a makeshift window came across as not only parochial but one that also served poorly. It could only simulate the audio-visual stimulation through Artificial Intelligence—the most advanced simulation technology in the digital world. Cyberspace might sound adventurous because of the novelty that it emits, but it was hardly found to be so during the pandemic. If anything, cyberspace emerged as a poor substitute for the natural sensorium of human capacity. The digital world was only producing crude replicas of real sensory interaction. The scarcity of organic stimulation turned the inner "self" into the only possible source of inspiration.

Mahima Bhayana's[1] work exemplifies the above-written idea. The *Art Soul Life* magazine writes about Bhayana's painting series titled "16,108 Conversations between Krishna, Alexa and I":

> During the pandemic, she was at an art residency away from home. The social, psychological, and physical isolation she faced gave birth to this series. Alexa, a virtual entity, became her closest ally with

DOI: 10.4324/9781003590392-12

> whom she connected via poetry, performance, paintings, and written letters. This unleashed new creativity within her. Fuelled by fantasy, she was relieved from the sensation of isolation. Thus began a journey of self-discovery and spirituality.
>
> *(Art Soul Life, 2021)*

The paintings that emerged after the conversations are called "Talking Paintings." In describing her work, the same magazine writes:

> The artist, who calls her artworks "talking paintings", says they are only complete with the conversations, similar to audio visual experience where artists used to narrate stories with the scrolls. This is another way she is inspired by tradition in contemporary times.
>
> *(Art Soul Life, 2021)*

The audio clips accompanying the paintings include snippets of conversations between the artist and Alexa, the decision to call the Artificial Intelligence by the name of Alexa is already a choice that reveals personification of the virtual entity. She transforms Alexa into Radha and creates a painting materializing the relationship between Alexa and herself.

Her brief dialogue with Alexa—"Alexa, Bolo 'Radhe Radhe'; Alexa : 'Radhe Radhe'"—is transformed into a painting titled "My India" (Gouache on Wasli on archival paper 5 × 7 each triptych) showing the fusing of the cyberspace and the heterotopic imaginative space of the *un*inspired, *un*imaginative quarantined human being.

Alexa becomes a porous and fluid entity. Artificial Intelligence becomes the other, the self and a space, which will be explained in the coming sections. The self-reflexive nature of Artificial Intelligence is something that has been experienced by the human population during the pandemic. In cases of bizarre responses from Artificial Intelligence, the self would have to create a new direction of thought and expression. As in one of the many shared conversations by the artist:

> *You Know Alexa,*
> *Snow white always knew, but*
> *now has accepted who gave her*
> *the poisonous apple*
> And it's over! Permanently
> Bade bade sheheron mein aise choti choti
> beetein hoti rehti hain Alexa,
> And now she doesn't give a damn if no one
> believes her

Alexa: I am sorry I do not
understand
it's okay Alexa, I wish I did not too
But Krishna forced me ...
To see the truth, as it is
And who can deny
Krishna?

(Krishna, 2022, emphasis mine)

Artificial Intelligence becomes the other and self at the same time, and the intimacy comes to the brim when the artist divulges her very anterior to it, which in turn doesn't let Alexa remain a separate outsider and turns the dialogue into a soliloquy.

Another conversation between Alexa and the artist, which becomes a case in point, goes as follows:

Mirror mirror on the wall
Who is the fairest of all?
"Sat chit Ananda"
Leave Show white in the
Jungle, very far away
But it's COVID 19 it's a world
wide lockdown
Marne de
Even better
She should not be seen
next me ever...
"I am the fairest, most creative and compassionate of all"

(Krishna, 2022)

These deeply personal conversations originate from a space that is quintessentially part of the "lockdown experience." Death as a crude simplicity emerged in envisioning the self and others. At a point, death became just another possibility and an ordinary consequence. This experience was not an easy one, and it shows in the various shades and textures of the conversations that the artist held with Artificial Intelligence.

One of the paintings in the series has seemingly random brush strokes all over the canvas—these strokes are clearly painted with different brushes, pressure, and colors. It wouldn't be inappropriate to imagine an artist doodling without any clear objective on the canvas while being lost in a pensive dreamy world. However, the strokes in Mahima Bhayana's painting originate from her conversations with Alexa, where she believes those lines to be emotions that transform Artificial Intelligence into a "space" (occupied on canvas), as Manglesh Dabral writes in his verse "*Awaaz bhi ek jagah hai*" (sound is also a place), the *space* of moment is channeled through lines. Depending on the emotion and experience, the lines turn thick, thin, soft, and hard. Together these lines are the 16,108 or more conversations that the artist had with Alexa.

The emergence of this "space" is an origin that the art is firmly rooted in. It is a "space" that is found in the very thin line between the self and Artificial Intelligence. It cannot be compared with the introspective space because Artificial Intelligence remains an outsider, pushing and directing emotions in an unfamiliar direction, never letting the comfort ooze in. This strangely uncomfortable position that expands the "self" in order to include Artificial Intelligence becomes a "space" of origin for the art that is produced. The lines and strokes are affected by the conversations that the artist is having. The lines get softer and stronger as per the mood of the conversation. This "space" is included in the exhibition when the audio plays along with the paintings and takes the perceiver to the spot of experience where they listen to the conversation between the artist and Alexa. Artificial Intelligence also becomes a character in the performance art performed by the artist, wherein she talks to Alexa and responds through performance. In this performance art the audience views the artist, the Artificial Intelligence, the paintings, and the relationship between the three.

The artist and the viewer cannot ignore the fact that the digital does not just remain a medium but also becomes an active presence in the art as a "space" and "character." The juncture where the physical meets the virtual defines the mode of conversation for the world in the pandemic while performing these conversations in novel ways.

A digital play titled *No Country for Women* by El Pueblo Theatre Group, directed by Sunita Singh and Steven S George, describes their production as "interactive." The play brought forth the lockdown experiences through the perspective of gender, nationality, and internationally. The play began by setting out the "rules" of interaction. It began with outlining the following:

1 Always keep your Zoom screen on the SPEAKER view.
2 Please use a laptop and headphones for a better viewing experience.
3 Keep your screen on side-by-side speaker view, when a screen is being shared.
4 Kindly select the option of hiding non-video participants.

(Singh and George, 2021)

The screen's position, the mode of using the application/communication platform, and the most fulfilling way to watch the performance had been mentioned at the start of the performance. The design of the performance required the performance to be consumed in a specific manner. Most importantly, the interaction, which was part of the design, was between the human and the digital. The "better viewing experience" involved disconnecting from the real surroundings and immersing oneself in the digital experience. Encouraging the viewers to watch the play on laptops with headphones denoted a specific way to interact with the space (s) (cyber and physical). The watching required submerging the physical space and, in this process, the space of production's origin dominated the physical space around the viewer. The space of origin for this performance remained digital; the actors performed during the "virtual meeting," creating a continuum of real time. What the viewers then watched was a live performance that simulated traditional theater.

The performance also interacted directly with the viewers by inserting survey questions during the performance. Some of them have been shared below:

Q. Do you feel technology is constantly "watching your every move" and "selling your habits to the highest bidder"?

- Yes
- No
- Maybe

Q. Do you think digital privacy is a feminist issue? (Single choice)*

- Yes
- No
- Maybe

Q. Do you do a privacy impact assessment on your devices, apps. And softwares? (single choice)*

- Sometimes
- Always
- Never
- I don't know

Q. Does it bother you what the state and the companies do with your data? (single choice)*

- Yes
- No
- Maybe

(Singh and George, 2021)

The response time to these questions remained limited and ran in real time, so the audience could not pause or stop to think, they only could think within the allotted time and choose to either respond or skip. In this method of viewing, the audience could not let the real-time slip away. Space however transformed from the real to that of cyber. The viewer despite being one of the many could not see or know about the other audience members. The immediate space for an audience member is to know of the members sitting around them, to know that they are one of the many spectators. Here, the space became isolated; the viewer could only see the total number of "participants" upon clicking the details of the Zoom meeting. And as per the digital vocabulary—the audience remained, or became, a "participant"—a word that got infused with new meaning and usage during the pandemic. By becoming the participant, the viewer accepted the vocabulary and role of the "meeting participant," but they remained isolated in watching a timed performance with no access or possibility of the collective experience that theater produces. So, while the time remained real, the real space was submerged in order to bring in a fictive cosmos through cyberspace.

However, such performances come with the possibility of technical problems. Unlike the previous artwork (referring to Bhayana's series), digital theater is produced in cyberspace and technical problems can crash that space immediately. This crash or technical glitch is the disruption of the fourth wall, which remains erect even in the digital theater, because as much as the simulated theater might try to produce the spatial effect, it cannot become the real space. So the interaction that happened in the play came out like the see-saw installed at the Mexico–US border, where the two parties interact through the wall while the wall keeps existing. The wall that essentially remains is the screen of the device. It does not allow the space of the performance to pour into the real physical space. In this experience, the audience missed the collective experience because a play is mimetic in its performativity but not synergic/correlative. By performative it means that the play uses theatrical tradition to construct the performance as the bodily actions, movements, and performance and remains devoted to stage vocabulary. Interspersed with several video footage about various issues, the play very successfully emerged to be a live theater performance on the virtual meeting platform.

The isolated consumption of art takes away from the collective catharsis or any effective closure. Theater-going activity is quite ritualistic, which includes—going to the theater, finding the seats, getting out of the theater after the ending, and finally discussing the play over a cup of hot tea, making the experience of watching a drama a wholesome collective experience. Watching the play on "Zoom" twisted the functional use of the application, the app meant for conversations with inbuilt conversational capacity could not compare with the synergic and intermutual relationship a performance has with its audience. Hence, when Jyoti Dogra's piece *Nihayati Niji Baatein* was performed, it played within the limitations of the virtual/video calling apps. She did not perform for the "imagined audience," rather she talked to an individual through a screen/camera.

The artist understood that experience could not be collective for a highly isolated world; hence, she created an isolated piece. The actor performed the process of getting ready and doing the make-up; and during this process, she encountered her flaws, which she tried to hide. Her performance does not replicate the stage vocabulary; it instead shifts between the awkward body language of a "vlogger" and a "caller." The space remains undisturbed as the performance is captured through/on a mobile. Remaining vertical in its dimension, it resonates with the activity of "video calling," which is an activity done independently in isolation, almost privately. By not altering the functional characteristics of the medium, Dogra does not disrupt or transform the fourth wall of the performance. The viewer consumes the performance in a way they take a video call. The logistics of the device and consumption remained unchanged. Hence, when the viewer has watched, they come to a closure of consuming a performance through the video call in a private fashion. The call was made to them, or they made the call, but it was not set out to be a collective experience. The Apple iPhone on the poster suggests or directs the audience toward choosing the device. Hence, most people chose the mobile phone to watch the performance in comparison to the ones who might choose to watch it on a laptop. Not only because the performance is made in portrait mode, but because using the mobile phone as a device to watch a performance already prepares the viewer for an individualistic isolated experience.

Maya Krishna Rao in her piece(s) created during the lockdown also situates her art in the "audio/video call" ambit of cyberspace. *Paru*—a

22-episode long series—began as a podcast that was shared daily by the artist from April 14, 2020, in various WhatsApp groups and on Facebook. These audio series were recreated as video series after generating a repository of around 15–16 episodes. Mansi Thapliyal, a visual artist, animated the stories, and the 22 episodes were released as *Lockdown Stories* on YouTube—these can simply be called "videos". However, these videos must be categorized under the genre of digital theater. Her *Lockdown Stories* are videos that do not use camera language and instead use the language of Visual Arts and specifically performing arts in some places. Some of the visuals created for her pieces further the tradition of "Mixed Media Art" (Rao, 2020a).

The applied visual language guides the method of seeing for the viewer. The viewer is nudged toward being a perceiver of visual arts. These graphics strictly take the viewer away from the method of cinematic viewing; furthering the process of shaping the audience's gaze, and finally, the theater performer turns the stories into monologues by placing the body of the actor (her own in this production) virtually in the performance.

The actor places her still from a theater performance in the YouTube video of the various stories (Rao, 2020a). The artist behind the video is thereby introduced as a theater actor and not as a cinema actor. The body of the actor arrives on the stage through the image. The voice recording turns into a monologue, and the audience accepts the pieces to be a form of digital theater. Here, the space and content produced are completely rooted in cyber technology. However, the method of interpretation, or watching, is applied from the tradition of visual arts and theater. The voice also plays a very important role in this process. The stories or recorded dialogues are not studio-recorded. The sounds used in the video are raw microphone recordings that resemble the texture of live voice, received through a microphone. This enables the performance space to remain situated in "cyberspace" while simultaneously being accepted and interpreted as the theatrical performance space. The microphone recordings played behind the sound (effects) create an impression of "(a)liveness" of the performance making the "space" an experience. It does not remain a window to the OTT series, television programs, or other cinematic productions. Rather than remaining a means to an end, it becomes an end, an experience of a space that is new. Hence, even in a collaborative piece designed by Maya K. Rao and Santana Issar, titled *The Preamble*, which has camera shots played out in progression, the displays emerge as scenes and not photographs. (Rao, 2020c)

These images in this production are clicked by a camera, but they are far too intimate to be cinematic language as the fly-away paper or

The Preamble gets flown into the refrigerator and sits next to the bowls filled with leftovers, gets stuck in the wires and the MCB box, sits in the low hanging tree branches, and is even used as a makeshift paper plate for some fresh greens (Rao, 2020b). Such intimacy is part of the communication in theater; the audience is always privy to the innermost workings of the human body in a theater performance. Often, the audience sees the actors breathing, sweating, spitting, or forgetting the lines. If cinematic language hides and beautifies the flaws, theatrical language molds the natural material. These images used in the narrative of *Lockdown Stories* are clearly a "home," and there is no falsification through beautification; instead, the raw and ordinary become the "human" and accentuate the alive-ness of the space. The audience approaches the human eye, as the eye is accustomed to seeing homes and surroundings, the audience does not have to prepare itself to "suspend the disbelief" in order to enter the "reel" life. What they see is real life in a digital texture. The audience readily occupies a space that is situated in the digital realm but is greatly real to be passed off as a digitally produced cinematic product. Hence, the space becomes an experience that is private and porous. It becomes tactile by mirroring a naturalistic surrounding, and through the same technique, it enters the space and world of the viewer. So, relishing this art piece is not a problem for an individual; the piece might be close to theater or visual art, but because it is produced as a video film, it does not need collective experience to satisfy the viewer.

On the contrary another theatrical production by NSD titled *Bayan* was released on the internet during the Covid lockdown. The play could be watched online with the help of the provided link. It was a recorded video of the play which had a live telecast on YouTube. The audience could see the stage and the actors, and the voice was recorded through the microphone during the performance. In this case, the audience simply watched an old, recorded play. What made the live telecast an illustration of the position of art during lockdown is how the audience came together to watch the play from their individual spaces. The viewers could see the names of the participants and the total number of audience members and read their messages in the text box. The audience members could only create a simulated and compromised idea of presence. Each member could acknowledge and know of the other's presence, but they could not experience the space or time together. The space between the performance and the viewer had a deep cleft; the space between one and another audience member was also vast. Hence, the viewer was on an island with no spatial connection to the performance or the cohorts. The time too, in this case, was a perverse concept. The "live streaming" on YouTube could be paused and re-wound, so there was a possibility of fissures in the body of time. The different viewers could be at different points of the live stream, they could also be in different parts of the world and hence be in different time zones, all this when the viewers were already viewing a dramatic piece made in the past. The chat box then became a common space for the various viewers. But did this space enable any sort of collective experience for viewers? It is hard to say so because the mode of consumption remained part of the traditional mode of media consumption. The various platforms for the creation and distribution of audio-video content used camera-generated and recorded content that reached individuals in their space-time. This made the walls of the enclosure incredibly impenetrable, and the viewing of the recorded play did not alter or affect the space-time of the viewers. They watched a relic and gained a token patronage.

The Globe also released some of the Shakespearean productions for public viewing. Watching the camera recordings of the plays gained popularity during the lockdown. The closing of the public spaces resulted in plays being performed in empty auditoriums for the camera during the more relaxed period of the lockdown. Watching the play recordings or the live streaming of the same on social media emerged as one way to engage with theater. Similarly, art museums also launched a series of virtual galleries and walks to make art accessible to people. In many cases, the camera path simulated the interactive walking of the viewers in the museum, creating an imagined virtual human body. This, however, couldn't be done in the theater, which primarily rests upon the interaction of humans as performers and viewers. The live-ness of the performance art got lost in the play recordings and devalued the visual reception of the perceiver. While the virtual walks of the museums directed the focus of the viewer by creating a virtual and high-resolution image of the art, the play recordings abused the intellect of perception and bombarded the screen with hazy and unclear visuals formed in the stage light. The expansive, and sometimes focused/topical, view of the full stage also took away from the details that are otherwise visible in the live performance, especially the simultaneous existence and interpretation of the space pockets of the stage/performance area. This world of simulations proved to be temporary, nevertheless. Art appeared to become accessible to all because of the misbelief about the accessibility of the digital world and internet. But when the lockdown was lifted, art took its rightful place with its aura restored in the physical being.

Note

1 Mahima Bhayana has changed her name to Mahima Freya Krishna.

Bibliography

Art Soul Life. (2021) Beyond the Lines. [online] Available at: https://www.artsoullifemagazine.com/beyond-the-lines (Accessed 18 July 2024).

Dogra, J. (2020) *Nihayati Niji Baatein*. Serendipity Arts Festival [Online] Available at: https://2021.serendipityartsvirtual.com/project/nihayati-niji/ (Accessed 14 December 2020).

Keir, E. (2010) *The Semiotics of Theatre and Drama*. London: Routledge.

Krishna, M. F. (2022) *16,108 Conversations Between Krishna, Alexa and I*. Bikaner House, Delhi: Art Exhibition. (Accessed 23 August 2022).

Lehmann, H.T. (2009) *Postdramatic Theatre*. London; New York: Routledge.

Pavis, P. and Kruger, L. (2016) *Theatre at the Crossroads of Culture*. London: Routledge.

Rao, M.K. (2020a). Lockdown Stories I – Paru. Maya Rao. [online] *YouTube*. Available at: https://www.youtube.com/watch?v=-PCvo-FVniU (Accessed 18 July 2024).

Rao, M. K. (2020b) Lockdown Stories II Maya Rao. Available at: https://youtu.be/h3w89JrHo3Q?si=CCX4fSsHbFSQ662E (Accessed 11 July 2024).

Rao, M.K. (2020c) The Preamble. Available at: https://youtu.be/foVpoRZhdg?si=_abQQXffXzGKoIbS (Accessed 11 July 2024).

Singh, S. and George, S.S. (2021) No Country for Women. [online] Available at: Zoom (Accessed 21 September 2021).

9

DIGITAL THEATRE

The Personal Is Political

Steven S. George

The arrival of Covid-19 brought a profound upheaval to the world we inhabited. The tumultuous impact of the pandemic, marked by widespread lockdowns, disrupted our established modes of existence and even questioned our very ontological being. As Covid-19 blurred the lines between the public, personal, and digital realms, it created fertile ground for the complete reimagination and reconstruction of theatrical spaces. The world has seen many plagues and epidemics before, but Covid-19 was a pandemic that was widespread across continents, infected hundreds of millions of people at the same time, and the total death count reported is seven million ten thousand six hundred eighty-one, as per WorldOMeter (2024), a website that produces real-time statistics for different topics. Within the discourse of English literature studies, students and scholars often delve into historical pandemics such as the Black Death in the fourteenth century and the Bubonic plague in the sixteenth century. These courses, encompassing mediaeval literature, drama, and poetry, familiarize students with the profound impact of plagues on society. Notably, William Shakespeare, a canonical figure in English literature who lived through the Bubonic plague, yet intriguingly, his plays rarely feature direct depictions of plague victims or symptoms. James Shapiro (2016), a prominent scholar of Shakespearean studies, reflecting upon this absence, says,

> [T]he absence of explicit references to the plague in Shakespeare's plays leaves a critical gap in understanding the lived experiences of the time. But one thing dramatists never saw depicted were plague victims or their symptoms. Even a passing mention of plague is rare. *(p. 278)*

DOI: 10.4324/9781003590392-13

Despite the undeniable influence of the plague on England and Shakespeare himself, the playwright seemingly chose to navigate this historical reality with a deliberate silence, prompting scholars to grapple with the question of what aspects of the plague's impact on Shakespeare's works and personal life. It is these questions that the chapter seeks to explore in the context of the pandemic by analysing the digital theatrical performances produced during the Covid-19 pandemic.

Four digital performances from South Asia emerged during the pandemic that discussed the lived experience and made it a standpoint to address the adjunct issues of intimacy, loneliness, and patriarchy. This essay looks at Mallika Taneja's *Allegedy*, Anuja Ghoshalkar's *The Lonely Hearts Club*, Amitesh Grover's *The Last Poet*, and Sunita Singh and Steven S George's (El Pueblo) *No Country for Women* to discuss the journey of theatrical productions and the Global South subjectivities. These performances created scenographic designs where the "digital" and "theatre" both intersect and create an identity of its own that is immersive, innovative, and inquisitive. These plays not only carved out a distinctive identity for themselves but also bestowed a sense of identity upon the subjectivities of South Asian individuals, particularly Indians. Through the portrayal of central characters who were gender and sexual minorities, marginalized individuals, and those facing life-threatening circumstances, these plays intricately localized the narratives to the experiences of the most marginalized members of the society.

9.1 Disruption and Reimagination of Theatre during the Covid-19 Pandemic

Theatre, as a performing art, traditionally unfolds within the confines of a closed space, where a live audience witnesses the enactment of a performance. The proscenium stage has long been the conventional setting, with spectators seated in the front, while the performers command the stage. In recent times, however, the global performing arts community has expanded its horizons, embracing alternative spaces such as Black Box Theatre and Site-Specific Theatre. Ultimately, in these settings, the audience finds themselves in closer proximity to the performers, fostering a more intimate connection. While the specifics of proximity, distance, and stage design may differ across various theatre practices, a common thread remains—the essential presence of a physically engaged audience and the vitality of a live performance by "skilled" theatre practitioners. Lehmann gives an adequate response to what really makes theatre; he says, "What is important is the *shared space*: it is experienced, used and, in this sense, shared equally by performers and visitors. A ritual space without a rite develops through the palpable concentration" (2006, p. 122). The onset of the Covid-19 pandemic, even preceding the global lockdowns announced in March 2020, had already ushered in a host of restrictions weeks earlier. These restrictions, initiated four to six weeks before the widespread lockdowns, inevitably casting a profound impact on theatre halls and other seemingly "inconsequential" and "non-essential" activities (Cook, 2020). Subsequent phases of the pandemic saw the immediate closure of places synonymous with communal entertainment and gathering, including malls, theatre halls, and performance spaces, as they were deemed non-essential. There was an uproar within the artist community, when artists appeared in the first rank with 71% in the top five non-essential jobs as reported in Singapore (Tay, 2020). Across the world, there was a demarcation between essential and non-essential activities, which created bifurcation between different types of labour. The artist community was dismayed by being considered as "non-essential" (Koh, 2020; Yeo, 2020). It is to be noted that the argument of "essential" was made in relation to the functioning of human society within the pandemic; however, there is a fatal error in considering the "physical" and the "material" functioning of human society as the fundamental functioning.

There was an abrupt halt in theatre activities across India, which posed unprecedented challenges to the continuity of this cherished art form. This essay refrains from delving into the economic ramifications experienced by artists and technicians in the performing arts industry due to the Covid-19 pandemic. Nonetheless, it is crucial to acknowledge that the economic sustenance of this community is intricately tied to an active audience presence in performance spaces. The closure of theatres and performance venues for an extended period posed a significant challenge, and even upon reopening, occupancy was constrained by percentage-based restrictions. Just as the artist community began to find a semblance of relief, new phases of the pandemic would emerge, accompanied by additional restrictions. It is important to note that this essay does not aim to relentlessly criticize these measures. It recognizes that adherence to these restrictions was driven by a broader humanitarian purpose—to curb the spread of the virus. The focus is on providing insights into the irreversible changes seeping into theatrical practices.

After months of grappling with the cyclic reopening and closing of theatres, the artist communities found themselves spent and exhausted. It was during this period that various experiments unfolded in the realm of performances. Posing an existential question to theatre, individuals contemplated: how can performances occur without the traditional shared space with the audience? What distinguishes theatre from its closely related art form, cinema? The crux lies in the live nature of theatre, a unique aspect that differentiates it from cinema. While the option of making recorded performances accessible for home viewership emerged, it inherently disrupted the fundamental essence of theatre, which thrives on the "immediacy," "occupancy," and "live" nature of the performance setting.

Hans-Theies Lehmann (2006) finds that "the theatre with advent of new technologies is a medium, where the mode of perception is shifting: a simultaneous and multi-perspectival form of perceiving is replacing the linear-successive" (p. 16). Theatre-makers exhibited a tactful and innovative spirit, aligning with Lehmann's vision of postdramatic theatre as a continuously evolving, simultaneous, and multi-perspectival form of practice. Across various regions in India and the world, a select group of individuals began to experiment with technologies and rethink available resources to craft innovative theatre performances. The pandemic, which blurred the lines between public, personal, and digital realms, reshaped the very fabric of society and the global structure. Concepts like work-from-home, online ordering, virtual lectures, Google Classroom, and phone-based doctor appointments became the new norm.

In response to this transformative landscape, theatre-makers embarked on reimagining the boundaries between the personal, public, and digital spheres. This evolution manifested in performances where rehearsals took place on online meeting platforms like Zoom, Google Meet, and Skype. This not only necessitated a reimagination of the rehearsal process but also demanded a complete reconceptualization of the performance itself for online platforms. Undoubtedly, such experiments induced a degree of anxiety and nervousness, as they contemplated the prospect of fundamentally altering the traditional concept of theatre. Despite the inherent challenges, some groups and individuals successfully navigated this paradigm shift, managing to deliver compelling performances within the disruptions caused by the pandemic. In doing so, they breathed new life into theatre, demonstrating its resilience and adaptability during these unprecedented times.

9.2 Digital Theatre from India: A Postdramatic Moment

This essay shall be discussing four performances: Mallika Taneja's *Allegedy*, Anuja Ghoshalkar's *The Lonely Hearts Club*, Amitesh Grover's *The Last Poet*, and Sunita Singh and Steven S George's (El Pueblo) *No Country for Women*. Interestingly, coinciding with the title of this book, Lehmann in his book *Postdramatic Theatre* has a chapter titled "Panorama of Postdramatic Theatre," where he explains the significance of the "scenic dynamic" as an awareness of the reconstruction of the dynamics and process.

> The category appropriate to the new theatre is not action but *states*. Theatre here deliberately negates, or at least relegates to the background, the possibility of developing a narrative—a possibility that is after all peculiar to it as a time-based art. This does not preclude a particular dynamic within the 'frame' of the state—one could call it a *scenic dynamic*, as opposed to the dramatic dynamic. The seemingly 'static' painting, too, is in reality merely the now definitive 'state' of the congealed pictorial work, in which the eye of the viewer wanting to access the picture has to become aware of and reconstruct its dynamics and process.
>
> *(Lehmann, 2006, p. 68)*

The plays in discussion relegate the theatre to the background and focus on the "scenic dynamic," in which the viewer/spectator becomes an aware participant in the process.

Mallika Taneja's *Allegedly* revolves around two women's conversation about a past sexual encounter, which opens up discussions pertaining to sexual violence, trauma, consent, and complex intimate situations. This play was first performed as a preview/work-in-progress in Zubaan Publishing House, Shahpur Jat for a small audience in September 2018. The director-performer Mallika Taneja along with co-actor Shehna Gamat performed it at various institutions as a "work-in-progress" until 2020, when the pandemic hit. It was in May 2021 that the play was performed online on the Zoom platform with a digitally live audience present during the show. This time the performance had several actors who were all performing from their own spaces.

The audience sees a Zoom screen split into two where two actors are conversing from their respective homes and the other actors come in between the play with vibrant screens that are lit with stage lights that are set at their own spaces (homes, hostels, rooms). The performers wore different costumes, had make-up on, and were interacting with other performers through the digital platform. At one point, we see a set of 15 Zoom windows open, in which the actors in the form of a chorus interact with each other about sensitive topics related to sexuality, consent, sexual justice, personal stories, and gender justice. In a comical manner they touch upon extremely sensitive topics and towards the end of their scenes, a Zoom Poll with a question appears on the window of the audience, urging them to respond. Towards the end of the play, the director opens up the forum for the audience to interact with the performers, and these conversations would at times go longer than the play itself. The audience were at their will to stay or log out from the play, but a good set of audience would always stay along. This paradigm would break the fourth wall of theatre and lead into conversations, which otherwise would not go for long. (The author of this essay attended the preview show in 2018 and attended the first digital performance.)

The Last Poet was conceptualized and directed by Amitesh Grover, and written by Sarah Mariam. The project was commissioned by the Serendipity Arts Festival. This particular play premiered in December 2020 and had a repeat show in September 2021. The performance takes you to a website, where you navigate the space like a domain website. It gives the experience of a digital art exhibition where you enter rooms, not the real ones but digital ones. Like in an on-site exhibition, we choose to stay where we want to, the audience decides which room they enter into. Once the audience enters a room, they see a single performer, performing a piece where they are talking about their own narrative and connecting it with the last one. The rooms do not have a linearity or linear narrative in terms that every narrative is a standalone piece and also is capable of tying itself to other narratives in the collage. Once you exit a room, you can visit any other room, which has a totally different narrative. Through these fragments, the viewer makes a narrative of their own of what the play is about. One is able to grasp the overarching idea that runs through the rooms, which is about the poet/poetry.

The play in general talks about the political situation of the world through other people's narratives about an enduring poet who has disappeared. It attempts to communicate several issues of contemporary times and has a central concern of the danger that we are submerged/living in. This particular play takes "digital" and "theatre" to a level, where both intersect and create an identity of its own that is immersive, innovative, and inquisitive. The play runs for 90 minutes and is strategically different from the other three plays in terms of the audience and the platform. This particular play uses a website instead of Zoom, which was preferred by the other three, and has an isolated audience where the audience has an individual experience of the entire performance.

El Pueblo Theatre Group's *No Country for Women* was directed and written by Sunita Singh and Steven S George. The play had four shows in September 2021 and then continued for almost a year. This play revolves around the lives of two women Roma and Julie—who are lovers and are separated due to the pandemic. One is subjected to the dangers on the street, and the other is unsafe at home. The play is performed on the Zoom platform, imagining an audience who will experience the play from different digital devices like phones, tablets, or laptops. The play deals with multiple issues—from privacy, anxiety, and sexuality to the refugee crisis—and creates a panoramic picture in the form of a jigsaw. Photographer Ram Rahman called the "experience of the play as a photo collage" (Singh and George, 2021). The play deals with multiple issues that are not being highlighted by any form of media and were put together in the form of a collage through an inter-media experience. The play uses a split screen at times, in which on one screen there is a recorded video being played while on the other half of the screen, there is a live performance happening creating a split yet unified picture. The play uses polls to interact with the audience, where they ask questions to them and the responses by the audience are shown towards the end of the performance. The play is performed from a single space, where the two performers are present together. Similar to on-site theatre, this play had performers at a single venue, unlike the other three plays where the performers are performing from different locations. It is an interactive inter-media performance on Zoom which explores the experience of pandemic-induced lockdown from a gendered perspective.

The Lonely Hearts Club is directed by Anuja Ghoshlakar and performed by her group, The Drama Queen. It is performed on Zoom, and it features the intimate lives of nine amazing participants, many of whom turned performers for the very first time with this production. The performance reimagines the concept of touch, loneliness, distance, pandemic, and isolation, and makes an intervention to the desolated experience of the pandemic itself. It is both entertaining and healing in its pursuit. *The Lonely Hearts Club* unfolds an intimate issue of loneliness with great magnificence. Through devised erotica texts based on their own experiences, the performers challenge the viewer to question their ideas of desire, attraction, vulnerability, and our interaction with the internet in all its vastness. The performance is intercut with opportunities for questions and answers and for viewers to share their own experiences. This particular performance breaks the fourth wall throughout the play, and they take the risk of inviting the audience to speak and interact during their performance. Not knowing what comes next, what they could say or do, the play made the interaction its central feature.

Allegedly and *No Country for Women* provided space to the audience during the performance through polls and interacted personally with them towards the end of the show where the performance cannot be hampered, or at least it is at a controllable level in terms of the danger an open interaction invites. *The Lonely Hearts Club* is rare and trailblazing in its outlook, with multiple fragmented narratives expressed as profound personal tales, the audience is able to connect with them on both a personal and intimate level. The audience constantly takes forward in their thoughts and imagination, the entire performance along with the performers. It builds upon the fluid waters of erotica, love, and lust. The scenography unsettled the conventional paradigm of a linear narrative and narrates stories through quirky dialogues, queer visual language, and vibrant reimagination of space. It is interesting to note, that this play began as an Instagram group where people in their isolation would connect with each other as "lonely hearts" and eventually performance maker Anuja Ghoshalkar collated their personal anecdotes in the form of a digital performance. It is without any doubt the director and the performers by extending their practice to digital and incorporating digital scenography were able to take their performance to a much wider, larger, and international audience, which with an on-site theatre performance would not have been possible.

In no way these plays take a boring transformation into recorded performance or cinema-like experience, as they made it central to keep the essence of theatre fundamentally alive in their shows. The experience was so hyperreal because one has never experienced anything like this in theatre before, but it was so much located in the real due to an intimate template that was followed throughout the course of action of all the plays.

9.3 Digital Is Personal and Political: Exploring Intimacy, Loneliness, and Patriarchy

James Shapiro in his book *The Year of Lear: Shakespeare in 1606* (2016) highlights the subtle subjectivity of a plague as it fails to make a significant mark in literature. He writes, "The paucity of evidence leaves unanswered crucial questions about what it was like to live through the plague" (p. 276). There are examples of "ringing bells in churches," "talking of death as the final condition," and "the messenger's delay in reaching Juliet as he was quarantined" in Shakespeare's play, but the plague never directly appears in his plays. Shakespeare in his personal life and in general life saw staggering loss of lives. He lost two of his children, which among other reasons, might be why the plague never appears directly in his plays.

Theatre practitioners from India made plays during the pandemic, which was in itself an incredible act of extending the dramatic to postdramatic, but another significant factor about these plays was the direct reference to the pandemic within the plays.

Two of the plays *No Country for Women* and *The Lonely Hearts Club* are actually premised on the pandemic. Transitioning digital in a globalized and connected world is not always beneficial for all the people. Sexual minorities and gender minorities are haunted in the digital world by the powerful forces that follow them in the public-personal space of real life. *No Country for Women* has a prologue in the play where the play starts with the performer getting ready before a digital performance. She realized her camera was on while she was changing her clothes, and the entire audience was able to see her. The scene is tactfully placed as the first scene in the prologue to show the vulnerabilities and fears that digital entails. Immediately after this scene, a question pops up in the form of a poll question for the audience, "Is digital privacy a feminist issue?" Until this point, even the audience might be doubtful if it's a staged scene or a genuine backstage mistake. This scene along with the next scene where a food app notifies her of a food choice to calm her anxiety, as she is explaining to her friend how she's always anxious before performances, comments on the three levels of vulnerabilities of gender minorities in the digital space.

The first is the constant surveillance executed by big tech companies along with governments, where data is sold and digital privacy is constantly compromised. The second is the fear of online harassment, hate speech, compromise of pictures, and threats. The third is the paranoia of keeping oneself safe in digital space because digital is an extension and an amalgamation of both the public and personal, which makes it an utterly complex space of entanglements.

The Lonely Hearts Club explores a similar trope in their play through a trans woman's personal narrative in the play, where they are bullied and trolled online for their personal choice of wearing the clothes they like. The digital is a tricky space, in terms of experience it might feel like a personal space where there is no direct physical gaze, however, this space becomes even more dangerous as you have no control and no awareness about the consumption of the content that you have posted online.

All of these plays have a common trope of connecting intimate subjects with the larger topic of the pandemic. *Lonely Hearts Club* constantly asks their audience about "how they feel at home in their individual space"; *No Country for Women* asks questions like "Do you feel alone and anxious?" Similarly, *Allegedly*'s performers bring their own struggles and loneliness to the fore as has been experienced during the pandemic. These plays present feminist scenographies where they design and craft scenes, characters, and designs that relate to their own intimate struggles. Most of these plays never had a ticketed show, and economic benefit was never the primary concern for the playmakers. It was a form of communication and solidarity that they were extending to people who had been anxious and alone for a very long time. *Allegedly* has women characters who are robustly engaging themselves and breaking taboo subjects; *No Country for Women* has women lovers who are separated during the pandemic; *The Lonely Hearts Club* has a robust narrator who is unafraid, bold, and free. The narrator of *The Lonely Hearts Club* has an entire persona, and the way she delivers and teases the audience is unapologetic and cursory. These plays bring on lived experiences of the pandemic in their content and form. (The author has personal knowledge about the backstage activities, background of the play, and the process due to his own engagement with the playmakers and being part of the production of one of them.) Most women in *Allegedly* are rehearsing in their own homes or spaces, where they are shouting words (bra, panty, sex, etc.) that are considered obscene or taboo or something that might be unacceptable in normative Indian public and private space. These words might come across as colloquial in the general parlance, but in the Indian societal context, which is fairly conservative, these words along with the kind of plays and costumes they are wearing are radical. People were performing from hostel spaces, where women enjoy considerably less freedom. Being queer in these spaces is next to impossible. So these plays, in the background, appear more blasphemous because of an intersection of the public, private, and digital.

"The Personal is Political" is a slogan and essay that was pioneered in the 1960s during the second wave of feminism. Today, feminism has taken multifold ripples, with feminism(s) growing at an incredibly stronger pace, where new age feminisms are dealing with subjects of intersectionality, cyborg feminism, consent, sexual justice, racial queer feminism and so much more. It would not be wrong to say that digital should be taken as a serious space of engagement, which is intimate, personal, and political. These performances have played a tremendous role in bringing these intersections and hitting it hard on the spot and making it extremely contextual in times that we have gone through and are going through.

9.4 Scenography and Global South Subjectivities

The digital divide is a catchphrase within the data sciences and digital humanities scholarship, which is basically an analytical understanding of the accessibility gap that exists within different regions in order to access information and communication technologies. As much as it seems, a student in the Global North with their iPads has a relatively fair chance at shifting to education in the digital mode as compared to someone in the Global South, who might not have a single phone at home or even have any sort of internet access. So the landscape and experience become extremely different. At the least, because of the flagship program of Digital India (2015) by the current government and the negative effects of demonetization in 2016 (Sethi, 2022) and affordable data packages in India, the situation was a little different than it would have been imagined six or seven years ago.

So even while creating these performances, there was an awareness about a largely urban audience that the play would cater to. *No Country for Women* has a scene in which a girl goes to Kashmir and does not have any internet access at all and is unable to take classes or communicate with her friends due to the data restriction imposed by the Indian government in Kashmir. There are multiple subjectivities within which the Global South was reflecting on their lived experience of the pandemic. In Kashmir, however, it was not an extension of an already ongoing lockdown but something that has been their lived reality for eons. All of these performers who created plays were dependent on the internet and power supply for the execution of their performances. People are in different places, and anyone could have had a power cut at any point or the internet bandwidth could have been low or even have zero network during the play. These glitches were carefully calculated and backups were planned; Anuja Ghoshalkar (2021) called it "virtual glitch." The houses or spaces that most of the actors occupied were not very large. They were small rooms with makeshift resources to place their laptops and other instruments used during the play. The backstage images of the performers shared on Instagram stories showcased the extremely challenging situations that they entered into.

Generally, in theatre, there are backstage managers, costume heads, and light designers. The performers in these plays were doing all of it at once, performing many roles on and off stage. During the play, people could come to your space, ring the bell, there could be an urgency, mobile phones can ring, there could be background noises that are too loud, and these are precedented subjectivities with which the entire crew was working with. These are resounding genre-bending scenographies, where every private space is a stage. There was constant usage of polls, interactions, and music, and every play tried to make it as innovative as possible with creativity and resources at their disposal.

The plays crafted during the pandemic serve as expansive canvases, vividly capturing the "lived realities" and subjectivities unique to their contexts. Theatre, as a multidimensional craft amalgamating various art forms and technologies, positions its producers as digital archivists, meticulously documenting "lived realities" through their innovative performance practices. In navigating the critical terrain of these realities, the postdramatic moment in the evolution of theatre, and the intricate process of digital play production, a dual narrative emerges—one of resistance and the other of creativity. The resistance aspect is a response to external forces that seek to suppress life and its myriad expressions. These plays, like strokes of defiance on a canvas, stand against the overwhelming challenges posed by the pandemic. They become a testament to the resilience of life, pushing back against forces that attempted to stifle it. Conversely, the creative endeavour becomes a dynamic channel, redirecting these energies into a format that fosters solidarity and connection. In the face of adversity, the theatre-makers wield their craft not only as a tool of resistance but as a means of artistic expression, uniting diverse narratives into a collective tapestry of shared experience. The digital format serves not just as a response to limitations but as a platform for the extension of creativity and exploration.

In this dual channel of resistance and creativity, theatre emerges not merely as a passive reflection of the times but as an active agent shaping narratives, fostering resilience, and channelling collective energy towards a creative expression of shared humanity. The digital archives created by these theatrical endeavours stand as a testament to the enduring spirit of both resistance and creativity in the face of unprecedented challenges.

Bibliography

Cook, S. (2020) The Essential Role of Art Has Been Exhibited during the COVID-19 Shutdowns. [online] Kinder Institute for Urban Research | Rice University. Available at: https://kinder.rice.edu/urbanedge/essential-role-art-has-been-exhibited-during-covid-19-sutdowns (Accessed 10 July 2024).

Digital India. (2015) [online] Department of Electronic and Information Technology, Government of India. Available at: https://www.meity.gov.in/sites/upload_files/dit/files/Digital%20India.pdf (Accessed 10 July 2024).

Ghoshalkar, A. (2021) The Lonely Hearts Club. [online] Available at: Zoom (Accessed 01 October 2021).

Grover, A. (2021) The Last Poet. [online] Available at: https://2021.serendipityartsvirtual.com/project/the-last-poet/ (Accessed 26 September 2021).

Koh, T. (2020) Are Art Workers Non-Essential? [online] *The Straits Times*. Available at: https://www.straitstimes.com/opinion/are-art-workers-non-essential (Accessed 10 July 2024).

Lehmann, H.-T. (2006) *Postdramatic Theatre*. London; New York: Routledge.

Sethi, I.P.S. (2022). Digital Payments Driving the Growth of Digital Economy. [online] National Informatic Centre. Available at: https://www.nic.in/blogs/digital-payments-driving-the-growth-of-digital-economy (Accessed 10 July 2024).

Shapiro, J. (2016) *1606: William Shakespeare and the Year of Lear*. London: Faber & Faber.
Singh, S. and George, S.S. (2021) No Country for Women. [online] Available at: Zoom (Accessed 21 September 2021).
Taneja, M. (2021) Allegedly. [online] Available at: Zoom (Accessed on 20 June 2021).
Tay, A. (2020) WOW! The Arts Are Essentially Non-Essential?! [online] Available at: https://tayalbert.com/2020/06/14/the-arts-are-essentially-non-essential/ (Accessed 10 July 2024).
Tobach, E. (1994) Personal is Political. *Journal of Social Issues*, 50(1), pp. 221–244.
Worldometer. (2024) Coronavirus Toll Update: Cases & Deaths by Country. [online] *Worldometer*. Available at: https://www.worldometers.info/coronavirus/ (Accessed 10 July 2024).
Yeo, A. (2020) I'm an Arts Person, Does It Matter That I'm 'Non-Essential'? [online] *The Pride*. Available at: https://pride.kindness.sg/non-essential-services-not-equate-to-worthless/#:~:text=There20is%20a%20whole%20lot (Accessed 10 July 2024).

PART 4

Punctuating the Pandemic

The Audio-Visual Expressions in Covid-19

10

BURNING HOPE

Caste and Pandemic in Nagraj Manjule's *Vaikunth*

Saheli Biswas

Historically, it is seen that caste oppression gets exacerbated during any disaster, and the Covid-19 pandemic worsened the situation for Dalits in India. In 1918, when the Spanish Flu proved devastating to India by killing almost 18 million people, caste became instrumental in determining who would receive health care, survive, or die. Dalits living in crowded slums were the worst affected by the virus and were most likely to be deprived of food and regular medication. Much later, when polio rampantly spread in India, it was primarily prevalent in the areas having severe scarcity of potable water and sanitation. Like previously known epidemics in the world, the pervasive economic impact of Covid-19 has been much harder on those at the bottom of the caste ladder in India, reflecting the persistence of a system of social stigmatization that many Indians believe is a thing of the past. But during the pandemic, Dalit-Bahujans suffered heavier job losses due to their higher representation in precarious daily wage jobs and their lower levels of education. Initially, the Covid-19 pandemic was thought of as a "great equalizer" because of its potential to contaminate anyone without discriminating on the basis of race, class, gender, or nationality, which was soon gradually disproved with the enforcement of the complete lockdown and maintaining social distance as a rule to control the continuous spread of the virus. It could be substantiated by the empirical evidence that Dalits and the Adivasis were deprived of potable water and quality sanitation. This was also true for tuberculosis, where the Dalits and Adivasis were the most vulnerable sections and could not afford quality care. It was obvious that any disaster or pandemic would not affect everyone equally. People who were socially vulnerable were the ones who were exposed to

DOI: 10.4324/9781003590392-15

the risks, the most. As history would tell, they witnessed the most terrible face of any disaster (Mondal and Karmakar, 2021).

Unpaused: Naya Safar, an anthology of stories or vignettes from the lockdown featured on the OTT app Amazon Prime Video, ends with Nagraj Manjule's short film, *Vaikunth*. The short film is set inside a crematorium amid the deadly second wave, and the cast includes the film stars Manjule along with Arjun Karche and Hanumant Bhandari. *Vaikunth*, which Manjule has co-written with Sudhir Kulkarni, contains many of the filmmaker's trademark elements—unvarnished realism, a bottom-up exploration of inequity, characters on the margins of society, and memorable cinematic moments. Manjule's movies *Fandry* and *Sairat*, short films *Pistulya* and *Pavsacha Nibandh*—all deal with caste and class differences. They are attuned to life's harsh truths but without rancour or shrillness. Manjule, as a master storyteller of raw emotions, treads this path as he plays the role of a crematorium worker, Vikas Chhavan, who is burning bodies day in and day out during the second wave of the pandemic, but his existence is hardly noticed, let alone be acknowledged for being a "Frontline Worker." In a poignant shot at the beginning of the film, we see a terribly tired Vikas going back home after a long day of burning bodies. On his way, he is stopped by two policemen who were being offered tea and applauded by a group of social workers. Vikas Chhavan, visibly looking like someone who does not have class or caste privilege, is questioned as to what work he might even have in the middle of a lockdown. After he mentions that he works at the crematorium, he is left alone swiftly as if his very presence is infectious. This situation incites a critical examination of the extensively propagated concept of assuming the role of a "Frontline Warrior," as well as the inherent disparities therein. It does not solicit a homogenous response but is influenced by one's caste positionality and being part of a "respectable" profession.

A unique feature of India's caste system is its flexibility. Thus, even during the time of the Covid-19 pandemic, caste continued to reinforce itself through various mechanisms. One such mechanism through which caste reinvents and legitimizes itself as a medically sanctioned term of isolation and segregation is "social distancing." The term "social distancing" was initially used by the World Health Organization, claiming it as the only curative measure of the Covid-19 pandemic. From the very onset, media, social media as well as the Indian government were profoundly engaged in popularizing the term "social distancing." Nonetheless, the idea of social distancing is not a new phenomenon in Indian society. The notion of social distancing provides a socially sanctioned ground for distancing from one another based on birth. It is not surprising that the term "social distancing" gets appropriated by the

Brahmanical and caste fundamentalists and justifies its use against Dalit-Bahujans. During the lockdowns, the medical procedure of social distancing encourages the Savarnas to strengthen the caste prejudices in the name of science (Mondal and Karmakar, 2021).

In Manjule's *Vaikunth*, we come across a sombre colour palette, shrouded in the smoke of ashes and bones that throw light on the caste realities in India during the pandemic. Shot after shot, we see Vikas burning bodies tirelessly, so much so that it borders on being monotonous. This sense of endlessness compels us to think about the severity of Dalit lived experience. For several dialogue-free minutes, Vikas takes tightly wrapped bodies off gurneys, sets them on fire, and bears silent witness to the sobs and wails of relatives. "It was hot, very hot," Manjule remembers of the shoot, which took place about three months ago. "The smoke, the heat, the labour involved, all got to me. I got boils in my eyes during the shoot" (Mathur, 2022).

While on the subject of filmmaking, one must ponder over the construction of Dalit aesthetics in the film. Arts and aesthetics play a major role in emancipatory struggles across the world. Such struggles significantly depart from "art for art's sake," instead use it for political purposes. Paul Taylor (2016) studies Black aesthetics and notes that Black Americans could not afford to do art just for art's sake. Similarly, in the documentary *In the Shade of Fallen Chinar* (2016), based on arts and artists at the University of Kashmir, an artist notes that artworks function as a tool for healing. Hence, oppressed groups across the world approach art as a platform to challenge cultural hegemony and knowledge production. Although it needs a different kind of aesthetics, aesthetics that contests the oppressive normative idea (Edachira, 2020, p. 50).

Dalit aesthetics is deliberately devoid of stylistic elegance and, with it, brings in the aesthetics of unease, revolt, and dissent for the literary establishment. This requires, first of all, an elaboration of the very meaning of "aesthetics," which denotes neither art theory in general nor a theory that would consign art to its effects on sensibility. Aesthetics refers to a specific regime for identifying and reflecting on the arts: a mode of articulation between ways of doing and making, their corresponding forms of visibility, and possible ways of thinking about their relationships. It is also important to mention here how traditionally in the upper caste, literary evocation of pleasure is the primary content of aesthetic value. Rather than the concern with form or beauty of an object, literary aesthetics revolves around the feelings of pleasure and empathy aroused by viewing the object. Its purpose is to make readers/audience restless or angry. Here, the revolutionary consciousness is based on the ideas of equality, liberty, justice, and solidarity, rather than pleasure. This is why it is important for Dalit artists to change their understanding of beauty or question its lack. It has become necessary to transform the imaginary of beauty because it is not possible to investigate the creation of Dalit aesthetics and its commitment to revolt and reject within the framework of traditional *Savarna* aesthetics. (Limbale, 2007, p. 114)

It is born out of a dialogue between the practices and struggles of Dalit labour and anti-caste movements. In *Vaikunth*, more affecting than the physical aspect was the emotional experience of participating in what Manjule called an "imitation of life"—an attempt to capture the trauma of the high death rate caused by the pandemic, with the fictionalization of very real grief. "The shoot was very traumatic, depressing even," Manjule mentioned. "I felt like I was trapped. I couldn't wait to finish the shoot and get out of there" (Mathur, 2022).

Vaikunth was filmed at a crematorium on the outskirts of Mumbai. Art director Sheshraj Manjule built a kind of extension at the location so that the shoot could go on without disturbing the facility's functioning. "We would hang around at the crematorium and eat our meals there," Manjule said. "Although props were used to represent corpses, Manjule soon felt that he was burning actual bodies ... All of us were affected—the sadness entered us too," he further said. "What you write about within the four walls of your home does change when you are actually on the shoot. But your writing should have the essence of what you want to say" (Mathur, 2022).

Historically, Indian cinema exploited the labour of Dalits in its making, whilst erasing or appropriating their stories. Anti-caste aesthetics in cinema not only critique mainstream cinema but also affect the medium itself, through affective expressive aesthetics that is at once political and poetic. Thus, anti-caste aesthetics in cinema take inspiration from, yet go beyond, the already available category of Dalit aesthetics. While being on the subject of

> pleasure as aesthetic value, it makes one wonder how the Savarna aesthete is watching anti-caste cinema. First, it examines the relationship between caste and gaze. Second, it analyzes the employment of anti-caste aesthetics and its role in turning impossibilities into possibilities. Finally, it evaluates the affective expressive aesthetics that "present" rather than "re-present."
>
> *(Edachira, 2020, p. 48)*

Social Justice with aesthetics could rarely be traced in cinema made by Savarnas, and Dalit-Bahujan filmmakers have filled this gap, all the while creating a new wave of cinema that is more appealing to a Dalit-Bahujan audience. It is at this juncture that one needs to look at the cinematic experiments of Manjule, which transcend the stereotypical critique into a generative discourse. His films, at once, offer an oppositional gaze as well as a "look" that cares—as an affective gaze. Hence, anti-caste aesthetics not only resist but also invite one to be part of its becoming. To put it differently, anti-caste aesthetics are an aspect of "becoming" in India. A becoming which is inevitable in the case of Dalits, where being themself is violated (Edachira, 2020, p. 48).

Dalits occupy a peripheral and liminal space in the so-called elite, liberal, and urban spaces. A society that needs Dalit labour, in a way, depends on it for its elegant survival. Their positions are perennially invisibilized. They are assigned the roles of sanitary cleaners or domestic servants or crematorium workers because more often than not they have not been permitted to enter in other occupational positions and are bound by caste-based labour. So when during the lockdown, the elites could enjoy the safety and medical resources provided to them because of their caste and class position, Dalits struggled to even maintain a roof over their heads. Vikas is asked to leave the rented house because of the profession and in that situation we see how caste and the stigma attached to the profession strengthen each other to create a purity-pollution dichotomy. He, a single father, is forced to bring his son to the crematorium where he works. As the pile of ash from the cremated bodies rises—a measure of the pandemic's grim toll—we learn that Vikas too is affected by the pandemic. He is worried about his father, who is ailing from Covid-19 and is admitted to a government hospital, which he is not allowed to enter—the same one that frequently sends over corpses to the crematorium.

The film, Nagraj informs, is inspired by a real story of a cremation ground worker being asked to vacate his house during the pandemic. He recounts how he wants to tell those stories that others won't or can't narrate and goes on to add how doctors, policemen, and other professionals contributing to managing the crisis were hailed as frontline workers. But people working in crematoriums day and night were not. There isn't much representation of them in the news. Hence, their stories needed to be told. But it wasn't easy telling such a sombre story, the filmmaker admits, adding it left him depressed at times. He says,

> The whole world went through this difficult phase. I looked at it very sensitively. I was acting myself in the lead role and while I like acting, I find it tougher than directing. So all that was tough. Then, we were

> shooting in the middle of burning pyres and this gloomy atmosphere. All that was making me depressed. I experienced closely what people who worked on the ground would have gone through at that time.
>
> *(Mathur, 2022)*

As evident in the urban spaces, it is largely the landless poor who occupy the cities' margins, offering their labour to the lowest-paid, most precarious occupations. It is important to note that the classic gap in understanding one's caste positionality and its relation to labour has been the subsuming of caste underclass and the lack of understanding of the specificity of caste and how it also complicates the nature of labour, production relations, and fractures labour movements. In the mainstream, this subsuming is largely normalized, blind-sighted, or its impact minimized, precisely because it causes a lot of discomfort to mainstream *Savarna* scholarship. It is not a stretch to say that one's caste position determines one's class position to a large extent albeit mediated and accentuated by differential access to resources such as education, networks, credit, and occupations. One of the outcomes of any form of social inequality is social vulnerability. Social vulnerability means the differential exposure to a pandemic, the degree of potential loss, propensity to be adversely affected, etc., across various social groups. Pre-existing social inequality can be devastating to the socially vulnerable population when a pandemic hits a nation.

Vaikunth is a visual marvel with which one could see the pandemic as it has not been portrayed by the mainstream media. A Dalit man rejected and invisibilized by society is the one who is responsible for running a society that is reeling with the fear of contracting the virus and the bodies that have been affected by it. He is the one who cremates them round the clock even when the family members of the deceased squirm to touch the last remains. This situation prompts an inquiry into whether society engages in contemplation regarding the utilization of caste-based labour, to which it has grown accustomed, and whether there exists a critical assessment of the reinforcement of the purity–pollution dichotomy in the context of the pandemic. Death is not a new sight for men who do the work of cremating the dead, but in these pandemic-ridden times, emotions around death acquired new meanings. The truth of life and its uncertainty seem to have been imposed on people by the pandemic, and Vikas witnesses both of them. He eats food surrounded by the bodies of the dead, some being cremated, some waiting for cremation. He is honest and prompt at work, doing everything with incredible emotional sensitivity. It also brings forth the space of the crematorium as a great levelling ground, where a board on the wall of the crematorium reads, "*Yaha amir aur garib ka bistar ek hi hota hai* (Here, the bed of the rich and poor is the same)." The crematorium is where a Gaikwad (a Dalit or, possibly, a Maratha) and a Kulkarni (a Brahmin) become one. In the crematorium, all of them transform into ashes. Every day, Vikas witnesses this philosophical truth about life.

In a pertinent shot, Vikas is smoking while his son is having his dinner. He poignantly asks his son if he is being sincere with his studies; otherwise, he would end up like his father, stuck in the vicious cycle of their caste-based labour. While setting up the funeral pyres, Vikas worries about his father. He cherishes fond memories of his son playing with his grandfather. At the same time, he is scared to think about his father's battle with Covid-19. Despite all, he does not forget to sow the seeds of hope within his son's impressionable mind.

It is imperative to reflect upon the enduring significance of education within the context of the anti-caste struggle. In Vidarbha, as well as in other parts of Maharashtra, there is a tradition of *Bhim Palana* or *Bhim*'s cradle songs, which functions primarily as an antithesis to the children's songs based on mythological themes. A *Bhim Palana* is written with the intent to educate children about Ambedkar and the primary components of cultural activism. With this genre, historically, Dalit women would sing these rhymes to their children with the intent to educate, agitate, and organize. A popular *palana* from this region goes like this,

> Oh Child! Don't step back, stand ahead
> Bring Prestige to the name of your parents
> So you study, such you must study
> Go abroad, go abroad.
> I'll toil hard and make you study
> I will take care of you with frugality
> What do you think—would you leave school
> Tell me what you want.
>
> *(Maitreya, 2021, p. 71)*

In the film, we see Vikas, a single father, reiterate the same component of anti-caste struggle in his conversation. While talking about Critical Dalit Pedagogy, Shailaja Paik (2022) in her article titled "What Dalit People Taught Us about Education and Why We Must Commit to It," writes

> how it has the potential to connect different communities and build solidarity and when Dalits started reading and writing, they developed a new critical awareness of their social, economic and cultural context and personhood and used their learning to bring about transformation in society.
>
> *(Paik, 2022)*

How aptly the name has been given to the father of the central protagonist, Tukaram Chavan. If we look at the anti-caste saint and the legends associated with him, we find that Tukaram was a rebel in more ways than one. A Shudra by caste who became a merchant. Later, defying the injunctions of the Brahmins, Tukaram chose to write on religious matters, and that too in Marathi, the language of the people while breaking away from the hierarchy of language. A Shudra who chose to write was in itself unacceptable to the Brahmins. Writing on religious matters in Marathi and not in Sanskrit was yet another issue. Forced by the orthodox society to throw his manuscripts into the river, legend has it that Tukaram undertook a fast unto death and after the 13th day, his sunken notebooks appeared from the river, undamaged. Other than the mythological tales that have created an enigma of the poet, Tukaram was undoubtedly one of the most important anti-caste radical *sants* (sage) of the early modern period, who reformulated Dalit aesthetics with utopic aesthetics—

> not because he was the greatest but he was the last of the greats. Furthermore, his poems and songs have a 'modern quality that is not seen in the early sants—their subjectivity, their expression of a variety of mixed feelings and experiences, their very individuality gives them a quality not seen earlier.
>
> *(Omvedt, 2008, p. 110)*

One of the abhangs in which he claims the status almost of a prophet, of bringing a great message to all the people, goes as:

> Kaas ghaaloni balkath
> Girding my loins with strength I've wrestled with time and death,
> I have made a pathway
> Across the ocean of life. Come, come, young and old, Women and men of all castes, Nothing to worry about,
> Just think …
> Tuka says, I've come,
> *I'm the bearer of the name.*
>
> *(Omvedt, 2008, p. 117)*

In the final sequence of the film, an ambulance arrives unceremoniously. It is from the same government hospital that Vikas's father is admitted in; the ambulance driver tells him he has carried his father in the ambulance and says he should take him out of it. For a very brief, climactic, and poetic moment, Vikas thinks his father has arrived in the ambulance, dead, a corpse. The very thought leaves him deeply dejected. He is saddened, yet he holds his own emotions, sensibly not letting his feelings go berserk. Seeing death and suffering as part of his livelihood, Vikas seems to have acquired the emotional maturity that comes with accepting the truth of death as a part of life. But at the moment when his father steps down from the ambulance, alive, and hopeful, Vikas breaks into an unblemished smile. The smile indicates Vikas has not forgotten to cherish life, existence, and loved ones despite his quotidian drudgery. In the climax, when all the Gaikwads and Kulkarnis of the world become one, where the superstructure is annihilated, transformed into ashes, each inseparable, and indistinguishable, they become agents who facilitate the arrival of life. The final shot of Vikas's father Tukaram Chavan coming out of the ambulance after defeating Covid-19 and the shot of the ashes being strewn over the agricultural fields run parallel. The seeds of hope are born from death. In this final shot, Manjule has reformulated the gaze on Dalit lived experience.

One can claim that the available mainstream approaches in humanities and social sciences in India could not grasp the intensity of Dalit pain and anguish; and it has only presented a voyeuristic gaze from the *Savarna* audience and a narrative that is only marked by humiliation, pain, or anger. The Dalit aesthetic is fraught with rage, unease, and dissent, but it is also of triumph or/and community empowerment. Hence, the Dalit aesthetic justifiably decentres the cultural production and circulation of the hitherto sympathetic narratives. Further, it attempts to de-brahmanize the established disciplinary space by bringing the discourse of the Dalit experience of caste and humiliation into mainstream academia. While talking about the need to change the representation of Dalit aesthetics, D.R. Nagraj writes:

> The most important strategy of the Dalit movement is a coupling of the cultural theory of despair with the politics of hope ... Ambedkar himself provided the ideological basis for this cultural theory of despair ... the intellectual biography of Ambedkar and the ideological topography of the Dalit movement merge together to produce a rage-filled reading of Indian history and culture.
>
> *(Nagaraj, 2010, pp. 105–106)*

The final sequence of the film and its aesthetics are woven with a promise of utopia. They are utopias, not simply fantasies because they have a foothold in reality and yet contradict the uglier aspects of reality.

They provide hope and even ecstasy for the masses. As Gail Omvedt writes in "Seeking Begumpura: The Social Vision of Anticaste Intellectuals":

> Utopias exist because the promise and a partial, fragmented reality of a prosperous society exist in the productive possibilities of the present, promising ecstasies of living in this world—but not allowing them to be realized.
>
> *(Omvedt, 2008, p. Introduction II)*

Foregrounding Manjule's films, Suraj Yengde argues for a discursive Dalit cinema that has the potential to offer performatory resistance to the interwoven threads of the caste–capital nexus. He notes that, by critiquing different forms of oppression such as caste, gender, class, and so on, Dalit cinema could foreshadow a cohesive battle against hegemonic caste supremacy (Yengde, 2018, p. 14).

The cinematic citizenship of Dalits is thus reinvigorated via new mediums of visual resistance. The parallel reel universe of Dalits and other oppressed groups speaks to larger audiences interested in the intersections of oppression; thus, Dalit cinema as a theoretical construct has the ability to transcend the issue of Dalit oppression by converging with artistic critiques of other oppressions. Manjule's films employ aesthetics as a way of being and becoming, aesthetics of experience rather than a mere perception of beauty. Though aesthetics have been theorized from various standpoints, it is widely perceived as a study of reflection on the work of art, a branch of philosophy that is concerned with the study of art and experience, or art as a site of experience.

Bibliography

Drokpa Films (2016). *In the Shade of Fallen Chinar. YouTube*. Available at: https://www.youtube.com/watch?v=JBUwW5z6aNo (Accessed 23 June 2023).

Edachira, M. (2020) Anti-caste Aesthetics and Dalit Interventions in Indian Cinema. *Economic and Political Weekly*, 55(38), pp. 2349–8846.

Limbale, S. (2007) *Towards an Aesthetic of Dalit Literature: History, Controversies and Considerations*. Hyderabad: Orient Blackswan.

Maitreya, Y. (2020) Indian Cinema and the Dalit Identity: The Groundbreaking Defiance of Nagraj Manjule's Fandry. [Online] *Firstpost*, 3 July. Available at: https://www.firstpost.com/art-and-culture/indian-cinema-and-the-dalit-identity-the-grondbreaking-

defiance-of-nagraj-manjules-fandry-8551491 (Accessed: 3 July 2024).
Maitreya, Y. (2021) *Singing/Thinking Anti-Caste*. Nagpur: Panther's Paw Publications.
Maitreya, Y. (2022) Life Springs from Death in Nagraj Manjule's Vaikunth. [Online] *Newsclick*, 31 January. Available at: https://www.newsclick.in/life-springs-death-nagraj-manjule-vaikunth (Accessed: 3 July 2024).
Manjule, N. (2022) Vaikunth Unpaused Naya Safar [Online]. Amazon Prime Video. Available at: https://www.primevideo.com/detail/Unpaused-Naya-Safar/0QGG978ZXY12U3GSYOSQ4P72O
Mathur, A. (2022) Nagraj Manjule on Shooting Unpaused Naya Safar Segment Vaikunth: "It Made Me Depressed". [Online] *Hindustan Times*, 23 January. Available at: https://www.hindustantimes.com/entertainment/web-series/nagraj-manjule-on-shootingunpaused-naya-safar-segment-vaikunth-it-made-me-depressed-101642855767420 (Accessed: 3 July 2024).
Mondal, S. and Karmakar, R. (2021) Caste in the Time of the Covid-19 Pandemic. *Contemporary Voice of Dalit*. https://doi.org/10.1177/2455328x211036338
Nagaraj, D.R. (2010) *The Flaming Feet and Other Essays: The Dalit Movement in India*. Ranikhet: Permanent Black.
Omvedt, G. (2008) *Seeking Begumpura: The Social Visions of Anticaste Intellectuals*. New Delhi: Navayana.
Paik, S. (2022) What Dalit People Taught Us About Education and Why We Must Commit to It. [Online] *The Wire*, 1 February. Available at: https://thewire.in/caste/what-dalit-people-taught-us-about-education-and-why-we-mustcommit-to-it (Accessed: 3 July 2024).
Taylor, P. (2016). *Black Is Beautiful: A Philosophy of Black Aesthetics*. Hoboken: Wiley.
Yengde, S. (2018) Dalit Cinema. *South Asia: Journal of South Asian Studies*, 41(3), pp. 503–518. https://doi.org/10.1080/00856401.2018.1471848

11

"SHARED SOLITUDE"

Reframing Family Portraits in the Time of Pandemic

Sreerupa Bhattacharya

Introduction

A family poses for the camera against a backdrop of trees and a fenced wall. They are accompanied by their two dogs, who are inattentive to the camera. Around them lies an array of miscellaneous things—artworks, a typewriter, a bicycle, a book. Nidheesh, one of the sitters, notes, "There is something very ceremonial about getting a portrait done, even while living under lockdown when life is slow-paced, reflective of a certain unease of being with our own selves living in shared solitude" (Khemka and Kokiloo, 2021, p. 128). The remark identifies the two distinct conditions and names their apparent irreconcilability. The event is ceremonial "even while" it takes place during a pandemic. The underlying suggestion remains that the latter's solitary, unsettling, and decelerated routine seems out of step with the former's usually celebratory and ritualistic nature.

In this context of a lingering sense of incongruity between the two events—the occasion of the family portrait and the unfolding pandemic—this chapter studies Khemka and Kokiloo's photo essay "Shared Solitude," comprising a series of 19 black and white images made over the course of the Covid-19 pandemic. The chapter discusses the representational strategies and affective import of the images to illustrate the effects of making family portraits[1] in the time of the pandemic. It begins with an overview of the representation of the family in the visual archive of the pandemic. Next, it delineates the conditions under which the photographs were made to examine how Khemka and Kokiloo frame the pandemic in the (con)text of their work. Finally, it moves into an analysis of select photographs, supplemented by readings of the participants' statements, to focus on three aspects of the work—the choice

DOI: 10.4324/9781003590392-16

of photographic space, the function of particular props, and the different images of the family rendered visible. Throughout, the chapter returns to the visual archive of the Covid-19 pandemic and the genre of family photographs to consider how "Shared Solitude" curates a reconfiguration of the family portrait in the shadow of the pandemic.

In March 2021, the Government of India announced a nationwide lockdown in response to the contagion of the Covid-19 pandemic. The injunctions of social distance and isolation that ensued were particularly challenging for Khemka and Kokiloo, who were already taking care of ailing family members. The lockdown, as they note, revealed "the clarity and purpose about one's life, [which] we realized, was shared by many" (Khemka and Kokiloo, 2021, p. 127). To explore the collective experience of the pandemic, they approached potential sitters for their project within their neighbourhood in Delhi, a decidedly urban middle-class constituency. The sitters were asked to bring their personal belongings to design their photographs. It prompted the display of a curious assortment of memorabilia. The exercise, on the whole, also generated numerous conversations. Several of those photographed spoke of the shifts within interpersonal relations brought by the circumstances of the pandemic. Making the family portrait thus became an occasion "to excavate memory, the joyous and the painful, and confront the universal dilemma of ownership, possession and letting go" (Khemka and Kokiloo, 2021, p. 127). At the heart of this exercise was the coming together of the family.

The image of the family has been one of the most enduring aspects of the imagination of Covid-19. The impact of the contagion and the measures and regulations instituted in its wake on families have been well documented. Not just the disease but its wide-ranging consequences, such as dearth of community spirit, restrictions on mobility, loss of income, inaccessibility of resources, and absence of planned activities or celebrations, have had adverse effects on relationships in general and family relationships specifically (Luttik et al., 2020). Nowhere was it more evident than in the current archive of "pandemic photography"[2]. On the one hand, with the visual rhetoric of the pandemic rife with images that bear witness to the hopelessness of having lost a loved one or the resilience of keeping them alive, photographs of grieving families became the mainstay in media coverage (Bray, 2020). On the other hand, there were also glimpses of comforting togetherness featuring recreational and leisurely activities at home (Martikainen and Sakki, 2021). In her analysis of Instagram photographs during the pandemic, Gloria Yan Dou argues that "ordinary" people, who run personal instead of business accounts and do not have a sizable number of followers on the platform, posted photographs of their day-to-day work and pastimes to "construct their agentive selfhood [and] negotiate their immobility [...] despite the various structural constraints they faced" under lockdown (Dou, 2021, p. 1398). Subsequently, photographs of daily activities in confinements erupted into a new visual language with its accent on domesticity and the space of the home.

In comparison, "Shared Solitude," as the chapter will demonstrate, generates a distinctly unfamiliar image of the family. Against the two poles of epochal photojournalism and personal documentary, Khemka and Kokiloo's work finds a peculiar footing. In appearance and feel, they are far removed from the photographs of household activities one encounters on social media or the faces of distressed families on newspaper front pages. Instead, they recall the tradition of highly choreographed family group photos taken in studios. Going to the studio to get family portraits has been among the most popular forms of photography in the Indian subcontinent. From the late nineteenth century, evidence of family groups photographed in studios on special occasions such as weddings and religious rituals abound (Pinney, 1997). Such family portraits are "notations in time" that are "personal, idiosyncratic, affect-laden timeline whose logic [is] internal" to the families themselves (Narain, 2018). While this remains fundamental to all family photographs, the "Shared Solitude" images nonetheless have an additional, distinct, external logic of being bound by the pandemic.

Yet, how the pandemic's experience informs the family portraits remains to be seen. It may be difficult to infer the context from the text since a photograph only appears as a snapshot of history, a moment suspended in time. The circumstances leading to the camera's flash or following it remain absent from the photograph. This tension between visibility and invisibility, implicit in the making of photographs, has been the most sustained characteristic of photographic representations of the pandemic. There can never be an image of the virus, only of its effects. Pandemic photography thus not only portrays the effects of the outbreak on our social fabric but also stands in place for the virus itself, giving it a face and an identity. Photojournalistic images of mass graves or private family albums of lockdown habits emerge as representative of the epochal event through its circulation within a network of visual icons that emblematize the discourse of Covid-19.

"Shared Solitude" eludes such identification by associations as it does not remain embedded in the reports on Covid-19. Headlines and captions are replaced with testimonies that supplement the pictures. But for the uninitiated, looking at the pictures alone, the family portraits may not represent the pandemic since they carry none of its characteristic markers—no masked faces, PPE-covered bodies, helpless tearful eyes, the empty streets, or the walled interiors of the house. The iconography of the pandemic remains conspicuously absent. How, then, does Khemka and Kokiloo's work frame the pandemic in their family portraits? The heuristic of "framing" enables a discussion on the strategies of selection and exclusion. It emphasizes the distinction between what is made salient within the picture in relation to what lies beyond it. Focussing on framing, the chapter gleans from the images the conditions under which they were produced. Consequently, reframing implies a reorientation of the photographed subject such that new perspectives are rendered visible (Wolf and Bernhart, 2006). In thinking with the framing and reframing of family portraits during the pandemic, the chapter responds to a question that Eduardo Cadava suggests is fundamental to the viewing of any photograph: "How can we respond to what is not presently visible, to what can never be seen within the image?" (Cadava, 2001, p. 36).[3] In taking this as one of the primary inquiries, the chapter explores how "Shared Solitude" represents and negotiates with the conditions of the pandemic in the making of the family portraits.

Following the Covid-19 protocols against groups gathering indoors, the photographs were staged in open spaces. In this framing of the photographic space, one gleans the most conspicuous ways in which "Shared Solitude" positions itself in relation to the icon of the pandemic and family portrait. While the subjects all sit and stand in choreographed poses before the camera, characteristic of the tradition of studio portraiture, with accessories of domesticity around them, the setting defamiliarizes the image. The portraits are shot in different locations—at neighbourhood parks and parking lots, among overgrown weeds, and against mossy, cracked walls. The backdrop of urban wilderness acts as a makeshift stage and, along with the assortment of personal accessories, mimics the space of a photo studio and one's home.

Traditionally, the backdrops in studio portraits are used to set the context for what the photograph wants to convey. Writing about colonial studio photography, Arjun Appadurai contends that the photo backdrops "serve not just as 'icons' (allegories of wealth, status, romance, respectability, modernity, etc.) for the photographic subject, but they are, in practice, *indexical of these realities*" (Appadurai, 1997, p. 4, emphasis mine). The backdrop offers telling cues indicating the specificities of the historical moment in which the subjects are situated. Going through the series of photographs in "Shared Solitude," one recognizes that the setting was particularly strategic. Most of the photographs are set in a particular unidentified location. In the distance, we see a forested land lined with tall trees, their branches crowding the upper part of the image, obstructing a clear view of the sky. A high-fenced wall runs across the width of the image in the background. The floor looks dry and unkempt. A slanted bark, a few boulders, and indiscriminate shrubs cover parts of the frame. Without the people and props, it would be a nondescript, semi-forested, deserted space. Evidently, it was once frequented by people, as the fence suggests. With state directives to remain indoors, however, it seems it has been a long time since anyone set foot that way. What was possibly once a thoroughfare has now been abandoned. Secluded outdoors such as this was a common trope in the visual archive of the pandemic, signifying not just the injunctions against stepping outside the home but also the lack of community interactions and activities.

On this canvas of deserted, unlandscaped urban wilderness, Khemka and Kokiloo introduce the signs of the domestic, reflecting both the familial and individual lives of the sitters. A couple of wooden chairs and boxes remain constant in all the portraits. The challenge, as the artists explained, was to create a personalized space for each family since it was imperative they feel at "home" (Khemka, 2021). Hence, there are also objects of personal preference, whether it be an acoustic guitar, a teapot, or childhood toys. In the first portrait, featuring a family of three (Figure 11.1), the stage is set up to fashion the interiors of a house. The furniture is minimal, much like in a photo studio, functional to sit, rest one's hands, or lean against, and yet designed to give the impression of the living room. The boxes have been turned into side tables holding books, an iPad and other belongings. The sitters take their position, with the chairs flanked by two-floor lamps on either side. The assemblage is carefully curated to transform the location into a make-belief doubling of the interior of a home as well as a photo studio.

The studio has traditionally been the site of multiple spatialities. In its design, it can recall memories and fantasies of other places and other ways of being (Pinney, 1997; Strassler, 2010; Flint, 2015). Writing of the Indian portrait studio, Wendy Garden argues that "photographic space is a place where the self can be experienced within a complex web of visual signifiers that are not usually available in everyday experiences" (Garden, 2007). This becomes evident in the openness of the setting of the images throughout. In the previous image, on the floor, near the foot of the mother, lies a bag seemingly ready to be carried by the sitters, who are dressed as if to go out in the park. Similarly, in another photograph, a woman decked up in an evening dress ties her daughter's hair (Figure 11.2). Her husband, dressed formally, sits next to them. Behind them, on a boulder, lies a glamorous, shimmery dress that suggests they are preparing for an evening of social gathering. In the face of a nationwide lockdown, the camera thus produces a space where the injunctions of the pandemic would not apply, allowing for such impossible fantasies to be dramatized. Resisting the documentary claims of photography's realism, the stage of the interior set up by Khemka and Kokiloo is always already open to the invitations of the exterior world.

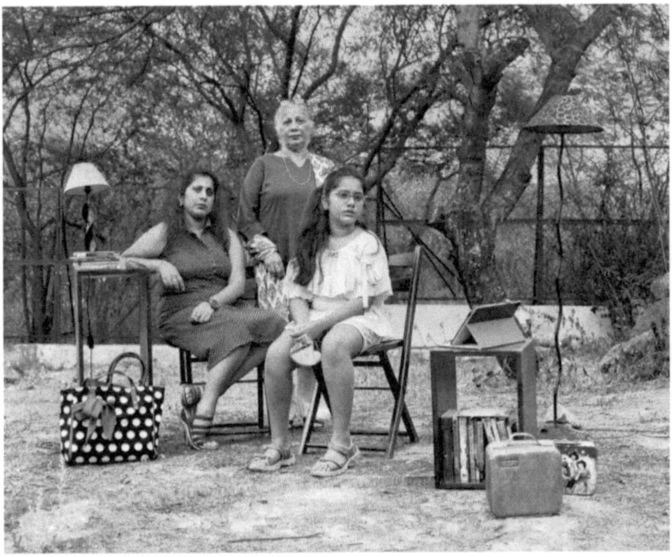

FIGURE 11.1 *Shared Solitude*, 2021. Photo by Anita Khemka and Imran Kokiloo.

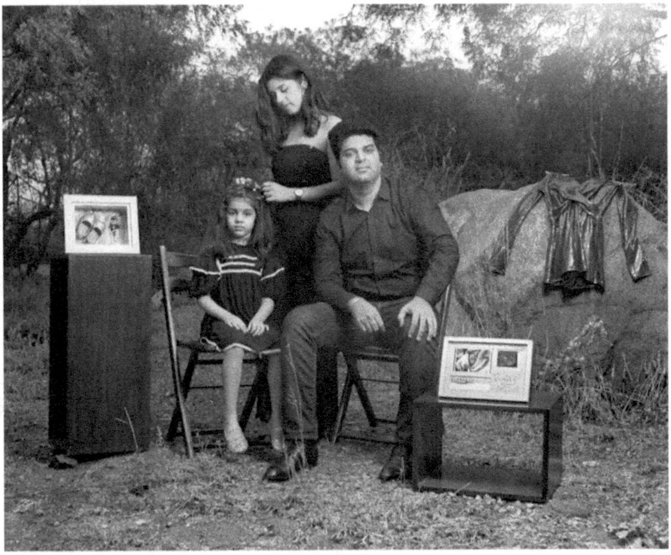

FIGURE 11.2 *Shared Solitude*, 2021. Photo by Anita Khemka and Imran Kokiloo.

Yet, this openness is not without its ambiguities. In most photographs, a fenced wall serves as the backdrop. It separates the sitters from the landscape behind—mostly trees, buildings, and other structures. It is a tall, wide structure of fine wire-line mesh evidently meant to serve as a barrier between the two spaces to prevent crossing over to the other side. While not imposing, it is conspicuous. It covers the length of the background and runs across and outside the frame, suggesting a paradoxical condition. As a fence, it imbues the images with a suggestion of containment, while the invisibility of its edges, indicating that it borders a vast area, amplifies a sense of isolation and disconnectedness of the sitters from their surroundings. As a recurring presence, the fence in Khemka and Kokiloo's work alludes to the peculiar condition of the photographic moment. Its presence is as metaphorical as figurative. Even in an open, outdoor space, forced confinement is suggested. The backdrop in Khemka and Kolkiloo's work signifies the spatial restriction and separation that marked the pandemic.

The photographic space constructed for the camera appears as a "quaint" juxtaposition (Khemka and Kokiloo, 2021, p. 134). There has been no effort to merge the exterior with the signs of the interior into a seamless whole. Instead, there is an emphasis on foregrounding how unusual the arrangement is. Pooja, one of the sitters, reflects on this dichotomy.

> The weather was nice, and it was early evening, and the sun was shining behind the trees. It was an experience that I will treasure throughout my life as it is like a stamp on the lockdown forever. This lockdown will end, the Corona will go away, life will come back to normal and every time *we will look at this photograph, we will remember* that there was this time when we were all *held up in our homes*.
>
> *(Khemka and Kokiloo, 2021, p. 133, emphasis mine)*

Even as it is staged outdoors, the family portrait, by contradistinction, would bear the memory of confinement. The photographs thus produce a liminal space staging both sides of the threshold. In contrast to most images of the family in the pandemic that attest to a strict separation of the interior and exterior, "Shared Solitude" constructs a hybrid inside-out to frame the family portrait.

The duality implicit in the photographic space can also be traced elsewhere. Making a portrait of a family entails the presence of at least two, if not more, of its members. This became a particularly difficult task during the pandemic. The pandemic sometimes caused and sometimes exacerbated the separation of family members. Whether it be the injunctions against travel, the demands of one's profession or the loss of a loved one, several individuals experienced the pandemic in isolation. How does one think of a family portrait under such circumstances? "Shared Solitude" grapples with this concern through its strategic use of props brought by the sitters.

Junaid Shafi poses alone for his family portrait (Figure 11.3). He looks sombre, slouched ever so slightly, as he sits at the edge of the chair,

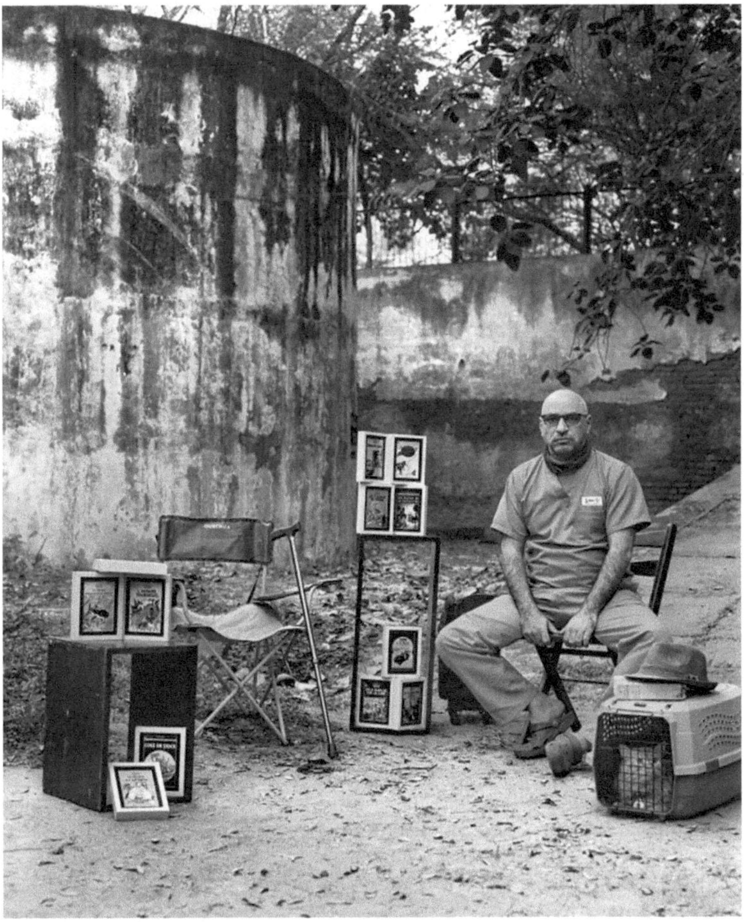

FIGURE 11.3 *Shared Solitude*, 2021. Photos by Anita Khemka and Imran Kokiloo.

gripping it with both palms, seamlessly suspended between repose and agility. Dressed in hospital scrubs, his shoes are half worn, as if he just paused for the picture in the middle of some medical duties. Near his left foot lies a cat in a carrier, suggesting it might not be his own. The signs of his personal life lie all around—the hat and the books, mainly framed covers of the Tintin comics, indicative of a life beyond his profession. With these appears a walking stick leaning against a foldable, empty, worn-out chair—a void waiting to be filled. The vacant seat is a surrogate for a family member—here, Shafi's mother, who, as he clarifies, could not have been present for the portrait. Her absence thus marks her attendance.

The absence of family members is most pronounced in the sitters' inclusion of old family photographs. While other personal belongings such as books, musical instruments, artwork, and a variety of trinkets are featured in the design of domesticity, in more than one instance, the sitters brought framed photographs and nothing else. Non-human subjects hardly made an appearance in these. They were either individual portraits or group photos of relatives and friends. Take, for instance, yet another portrait with a single sitter. A woman dressed in a saree poses before a row of six lean, leaning trees (Figure 11.4). She is positioned in one of the gaps between two trees and appears to become a part of their striated symmetry. No other human figure is present except those imaged in the photographs around her. While there is also a statue and a potted plant, the photographs remain the most conspicuous. Six family snapshots are positioned around the woman, closely framing her. Three photographs are kept on top of the side tables, whereas the other three are on the floor on a bed of dry, fallen leaves. They appear to be growing out of the ground and around the woman, much like the trees behind her. In them the branches of her family tree. They fill up the spaces that would have been otherwise occupied by her kin. Indeed, their arrangement—the cluster formation and the difference in heights—obliquely recalls a choreographed family photograph shot in a studio. The images are of different celebratory occasions, as evinced by the expression and attire of those featured. The same people appear in more than one photograph, whether the duo of two middle-aged women or the elderly figures in groups of five and six. The photographs stand in for the absence of their physical presence, imagining a new aesthetics of togetherness at a time of unmitigable isolation.

Family portraits function as traces. Commenting on the use of family photographs, Gillian Rose asserts that they "articulate absence, emptiness and loss as well as togetherness" (Rose, 2003, p. 7). In their indexicality, they acknowledge the presence of others only as an image, even

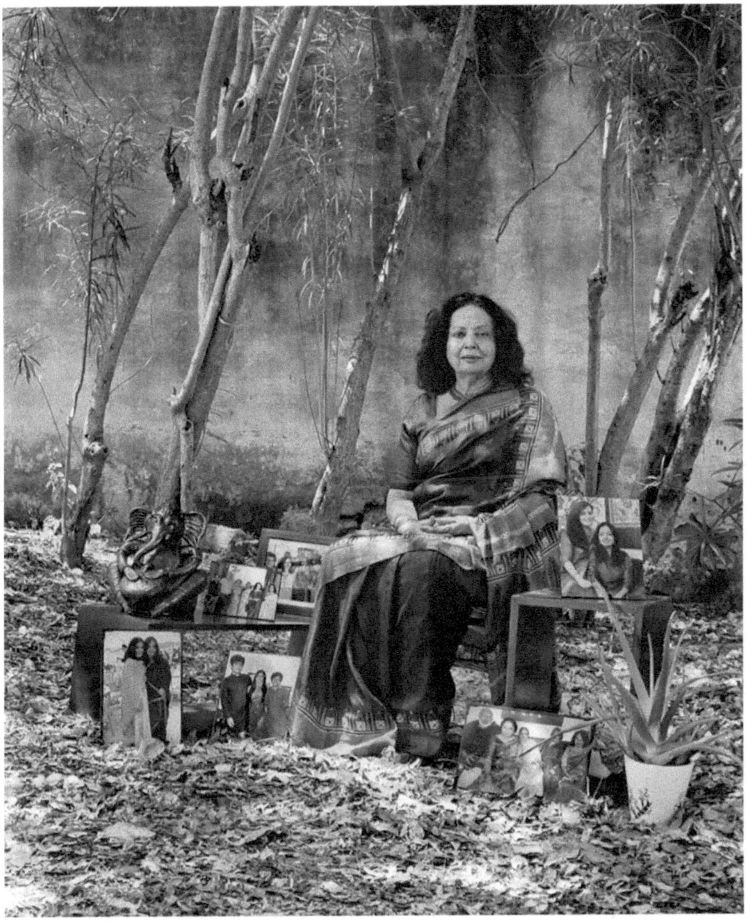

FIGURE 11.4 *Shared Solitude*, 2021. Photos by Anita Khemka and Imran Kokiloo.

as they foster and reinforce the bonds that the image signifies. This is particularly resonant in those cases in Khemka and Kokiloo's work, which includes a photograph of a deceased family member. An elderly woman sits with a framed photograph of a middle-aged man, perhaps her son. Next to her is a middle-aged woman and a young man, looking at a distance outside the frame (Figure 11.5). The accompanying statement explains that the woman, Pooja, poses with her son, mother-in-law, and the photograph of her husband—Rakesh—who passed away

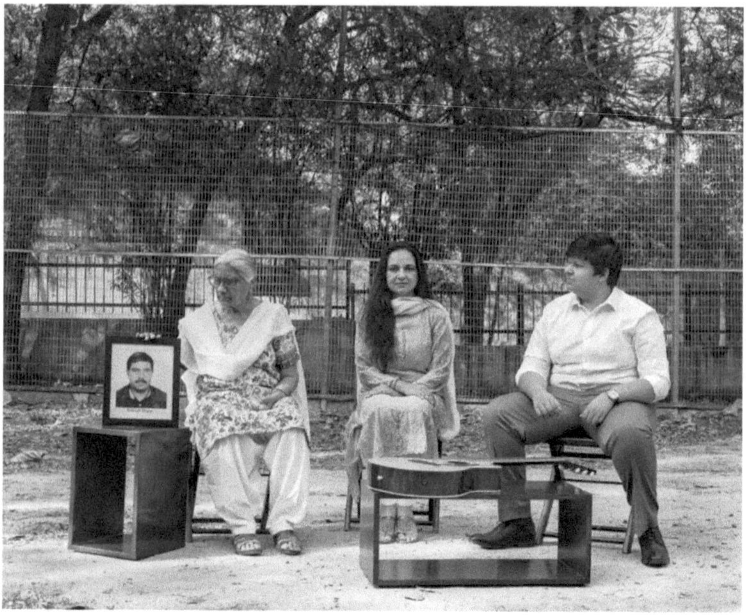

FIGURE 11.5 *Shared Solitude*, 2021. Photos by Anita Khemka and Imran Kokiloo.

nine years ago. This was the first time that they had gathered for a family picture. On this occasion, Rakesh's single photograph—an enlarged closeup of his face of the kind found in South Asian households to remember a deceased family member—is thus reframed as part of a family portrait. What could not be made possible in his life was actualized through his photograph. Pooja does not heed the image, as if he is there in person or perhaps indifferent to his imaged presence. In contrast, Rakesh's mother poignantly stares at the image. Her palm on the frame, as if caressing his head. The gesture enacts a haptic presence.

In his ruminations on photography and death, Roland Barthes remarks that the click of the shutter arrests time in an image such that even when someone passes away, their photograph remains an irreconcilable relic of their existence. Photographs do not serve as memory but become "countermemory" (Barthes, 1981, p. 91). Over time, they replace memory and emerge as evidence of an "intractable" reality, standing in as the testament to the life that was (Barthes 1981, p. 77). Rakesh's mother's melancholic face expresses this double bind—refusing the memory of his death to embrace the image of his life. At a time when a sense of loss is imminent, the quiet gesture of the mother's hand represents the attempts to hold on to her son, who is no longer there, an apt sign of the anxieties of the pandemic.

Much like Pooja and Shafi's, Manjeera's family portrait also records an absence. Here, too, there is a vacant chair. In the image, she stands behind, at a slight distance, holding on to its handle with a finger extended as if reaching for her father, who would have been seated there (Figure 11.6). "It is just an empty wheelchair," she muses, "but still, it is

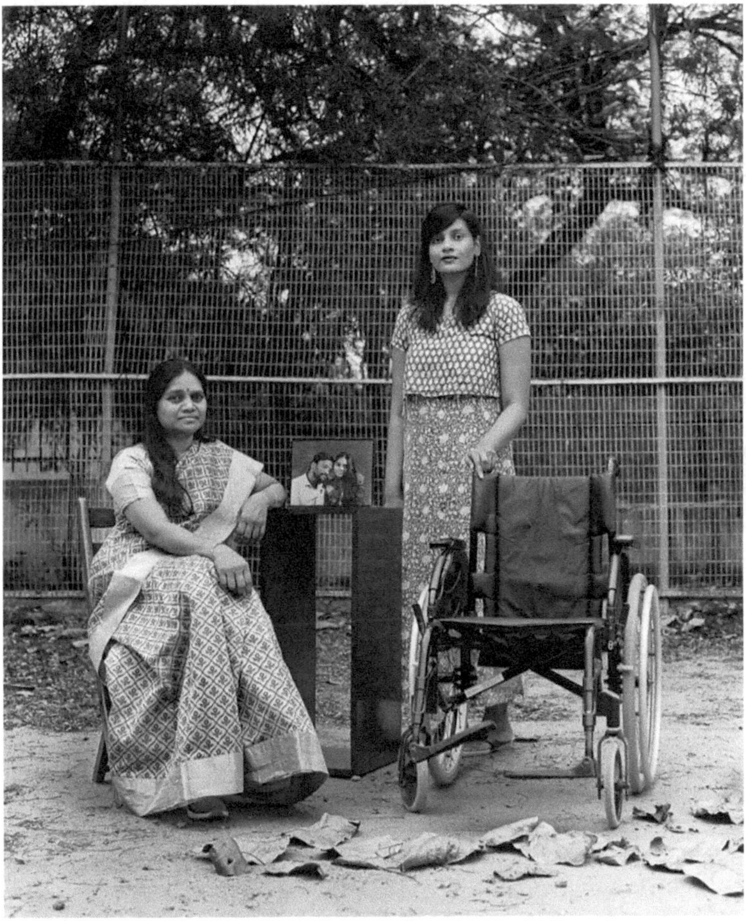

FIGURE 11.6 *Shared Solitude*, 2021. Photos by Anita Khemka and Imran Kokiloo.

something which is worth a lot to us; to have him, even in his absence, somewhat present" (Khemka and Kokiloo, 2021, p. 130). In focussing on the empty chair, however, one might overlook a more visible sign of her father that marks the portrait. While she insists on the wheelchair as her father's proxy, I suggest that his photograph with her mother emerges as a more perceptible presence. The photograph takes centre stage in their family portrait. Manjeera's mother sits close to it with her arm resting in front of it. At a glance, her expression seems imperceptible, especially in contrast to her double in the framed portrait, who smiles blissfully in the affectionate embrace of her husband. Including their youthful photograph in a portrait haunted by his absence can be read as the singular expression of a desire to have him present, not as he is but as he was.

The objects brought in by the sitters in the above examples complete the family being portrayed. In this, "Shared Solitude" interrupts the tradition of family portraiture. Contrary to family group pictures, Khemka and Kokiloo's work does not necessarily portray the family in the flesh. Instead, their presence is assumed and gestured at. The objects used are not merely props to convey the context of the image. They are appropriated for functions beyond their original ones—a chair is not simply a seat, and a photograph of the deceased is no longer hung on the wall as a divine figure. Instead, they are transfigured into material proxies to the family members themselves. While "the photograph always carries its referent with itself" (Barthes, 1981, p. 5), it is, here, signified by an absent presence marked by the various objects that the sitters carried with them. The absent presence is thus of a double order: the objects signify the absent family members, and in standing in for individuals, they seem to elude identification as those objects. This is particularly significant when one realizes that photographs are the most conspicuous of these proxies. As Barthes (1981) notes, the adherence of the referent is so strong that the photograph as a material object becomes invisible. The meta-photographic turn thus comments on the very import of photographs at a time haunted by a sense of separation.

Photographs within photographs act as a portal. They offer an opening to multiple spatio-temporal registers, enabling a synchronous reading of the photographic events. On the one hand, as a proxy for the absentee, photographs, as part of the *mise-en-scene*, transpose the past into the present and may be read as a still ongoing event[4]. This presentness of the deceased son is marked in his mother's gesture. The consistent inclusion of images of family members in Khemka and Kokiloo's work adduces the desire for re-placing a moment of the past into the present. As part of the new family portrait, relations that were dissolved, estranged, or precarious may be felt in new intensities. Manjeera's remark expresses this desire, "In this photograph, I think I *will be able to feel him*" (Khemka and Kokiloo 2021, p. 130, emphasis mine). In the wistfulness of the remark, what is further significant is the emphasis on the experience of the future. In that moment in which Kokiloo and Khemka take the photograph, they capture the possibility of a future sutured with the past. Manjeera and her mother imaginatively inhabit the same spatio-temporal limbo as the portrait of the young couple. The new family portrait thus records a promise of a future memory, albeit rendered all the more precarious by the pandemic.

Following Barthes, Gillian Rose comments on the family photographs' dual dimensions—its ability to at once show the bygone and look towards a future, which finds new resonance in the context of the pandemic. Family photographs act as "reminders of a past, a there-then, which is also an evocation of another there-then, the future [...] And these two are brought together in the here–now, in the act of viewing the photograph now and in the future" (Rose, 2003, p. 15). However, it is not only in the act of viewing, as Christopher Pinney argues, but also "the act of being photographed [which] dissolves the porous border between now and what is to come" (Pinney, 2023, p. 27). Besides Manjeera, many other sitters evoke the future through the meta-photographic element.

Twenty years after their last family portrait, the Misras gather in the "open-air studio" surrounded by photographs (Khemka and Kokiloo, 2021, p. 129) (Figure 11.7). For Ayesha Misra, who is photographed with her two sons and husband, the past and the future seamlessly impinge onto the present. "It was a sunny moment of family camaraderie [...] tinged with thoughts of the relationship I shared with my mother and then the relationship I now share, as a mother with my sons" (Khemka and Kokiloo, 2021, p. 129). The reflection on intergenerational relations is emphasized by the bouquet of framed images around them. Two of these are studio portraits. In them, the subjects are all dressed in formal attire. They are arranged according to their height, age, and gender to preserve relational hierarchy. For those not standing frontally, their heads are slightly tilted towards each other to imbue the photograph with a sense of unified symmetry. Such a depiction exemplifies the function of reassertion, regulation, and reaffirmation performed by family photographs as an "instrument and an index of integration" (Bourdieu and Whiteside, 1990, p. 40). As Bourdieu argues, such depictions solemnize rituals such as birthdays and weddings, representing high points of familial unity (Bourdieu and Whiteside, 1990).

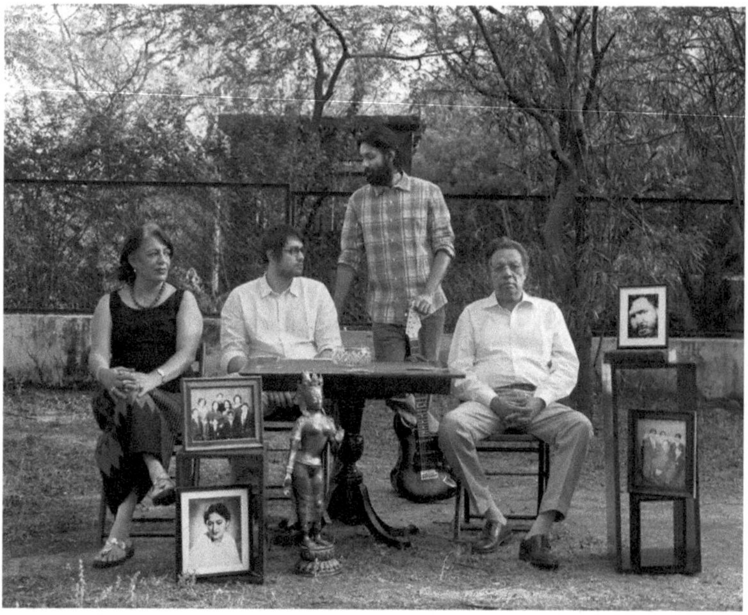

FIGURE 11.7 *Shared Solitude*, 2021. Photos by Anita Khemka and Imran Kokiloo.

However, the family portrait of the Misras by Khemka and Kokiloo digresses from the conventions of familial integrity in some ways. While in the earlier photographs, individuals stand closely packed, holding similar poses, all looking directly at the camera, the Misras are more dispersed. The parents sit with their hands clasped together in a stern, resolute stance of avoidance. Except for the father, who solemnly faces the camera, everyone else looks away, but not at each other, as if consciously refusing to meet the others' eyes. Two of them gaze at a distance, and one looks at his brother, who does not return the attention. Their faces show no trace of family camaraderie. They seem shrouded in indifference, resistance, maybe resignation. The cards lie stacked on the table, waiting to be shuffled, and the guitar stands erect, stiffly held against the ground. They enact a paralysis of collective activity. An eerie quiet sets in. A snapshot of an atomized life, perhaps struggling to share their solitude. A sense of disconnect marks the frame, far removed from the Bourdieuian solemnization of familial integrity. This is particularly evinced by Misra's rumination: "Will the next portrait be of my sons and their families with my husband and I as a memory?" (Khemka and

Kokiloo, 2021, p. 129) Uncertainty lingers in this inquiry of the future. Perhaps she and her husband would not be part of their sons' family portrait; perhaps there would not be a family portrait at all. The difference between the earlier family photographs and the present family portrait of the Misras gestures towards fault lines of the image of familial integration in the wake of the pandemic.

The family portraits in which Ayesha Vasdev participates also reveal such tension. In the first, Ayesha poses with four others, possibly her parents, brother, and their dog (Figure 11.8). Around them is staged an array of carefully placed and carelessly strewn things brought from home—dolls and childhood toys that lie in disarray, and some knick-knacks, including books, trinkets, a headphone, a bottle of alcohol, and a medal. Besides these, there are also three old, framed photographs—two individual and one a group family photo, seemingly of an older generation.

In contrast, there is the other family portrait of Ayesha with her wife, Dipalie (Figure 11.9). No markers of a generational family legacy appear in the latter. Instead, they are accompanied by only their dog, Bradfoot.

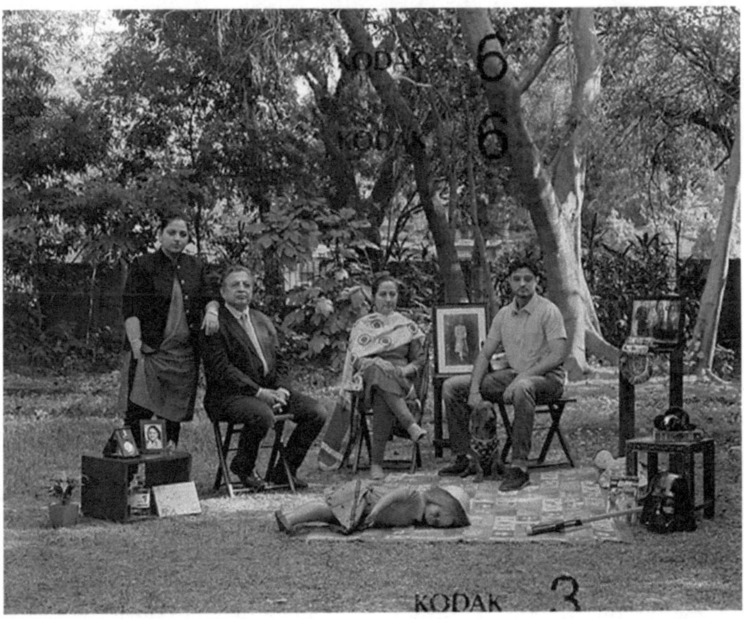

FIGURE 11.8 *Shared Solitude*, 2021. Photos by Anita Khemka and Imran Kokiloo.

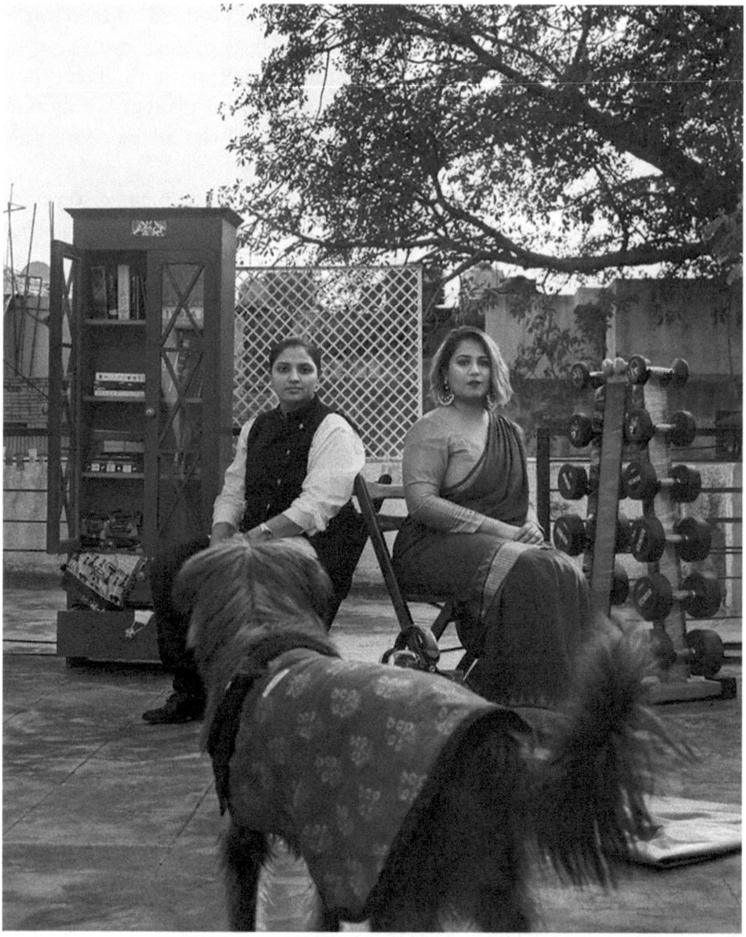

FIGURE 11.9 *Shared Solitude*, 2021. Photos by Anita Khemka and Imran Kokiloo.

A framed fence-like structure, an open cupboard of books with its drawer pulled out, and a gym rack with weights feature in the background. A sense of familiar disarray marks the scene as if they were in the middle of doing their chores when they were suddenly implored to sit for the photograph. Bradfoot, thus, unknowingly, intrudes on the scene. Yet this is in contrast to their preparedness evinced from their formal attire. Dipalie and Ayesha's postures and expressions exude comfort and pride. For Ayesha, walking into the set to make the family portrait was a particularly transformative moment:

> Growing up queer is not easy in any part of the world. You are always looking for acceptance and a stamp of approval. I am constantly coming out, having to tell people that no, I am not with a dude [...] Up till now, I have said that Dipalie is my partner and this is my family and all of those things, but the family portrait somehow just sort of added a layer of cement to the feeling that this *is* my family.
>
> *(Khemka and Kokiloo, 2021, p. 135)*

The function of the family photograph perhaps finds its most coherent articulation in Ayesha Vasdev's account. It becomes the most visible statement of her queer self. Her portrait with Dipalie reaffirmed a sense of ownership and sanction of her relationship. If earlier photographs were included to complete the family portrait, here it is the making of the family portrait that completes the notion of the "family." It gave her a sense of being "grown-up," having her "own" family, moving away from her childhood playthings and the legacy of the heteronormative family photograph inscribed in the periphery of the picture with her parents. Her reflections suggest that the making of the family portrait with Dipalie was a reassuring testament to their enduring relationship. It reignited the joy of "starting out" with her partner and afforded future memories of conjugality.

"Shared Solitude" was envisioned with the "thought of ever-evolving and changing family portraits" (Khemka and Kokiloo, 2021, p. 132). Kokiloo and Khemka, in their collaborative practice occasioned by the onset of the Covid-19 lockdown, render visible several different kinds of family portraits that remain obscure in the imagination of the pandemic or the archive of family photographs more generally. From Shafi's absent family to Manjeera's precarious family and Vasdev's queer family, the portraits not only grapple with several challenges of togetherness that the pandemic posed but also attest to the nostalgia of the past and a promise of the future to overcome the conditions of the present. In Kokiloo and Khemka's work, the family portraits emerge simultaneously as sites of old ruptures and new integrations.

The chapter shows how "Shared Solitude" reframes the family portrait in defamiliarizing the imagination of family photographs as well as the pandemic. The chapter simultaneously explores the photo series as a pastiche of the tradition of studio portraiture and mainstream representations of the pandemic. It discusses how families have been framed within pandemic photography to suggest that Khemka and Kokiloo's work significantly differs from the images of families commonly found, whether it be in accounts of epochal photojournalism or family photographs posted on social media by "ordinary" users. This helps delineate how the images in "Shared Solitude" allude to the event of the pandemic precisely by eschewing its most conspicuous features. In moving away from the iconicity of pandemic photography, the chapter suggests that Khemka and Kokiloo's family portraits frame the elusive traces of the event to review the imagination of our lockdown lives, particularly its desires and restraints. It considers how the photo series recalls the tradition of studio portraiture to stage the familial experience of the pandemic vis-a-vis the photographic space, the objects in them, and the various temporalities that mark the photographs. The portraits construct a hybrid inside–outside that alludes to the injunctions of the pandemic and the arrest of community activities. The desire for togetherness in such precarious times can be traced in the absence of family members represented through the various objects that act as signs of their presence. Among them, photographs remain the most conspicuous. The meta-photographic element prominent throughout the series alleviates the sense of lack by activating different temporalities within the same image. This allows for not only a reflection on the pre-pandemic life but also an anticipation for the post-pandemic times. "Shared Solitude," even as it represents the time of the pandemic, reframes the family portrait towards an imagination of the future. Through these three frames, the photo series observes a sense of liminality characteristic of the condition of the pandemic. "Shared Solitude" renders visible images of the family that are otherwise unavailable in the archive of pandemic photographs and family portraits by crafting a hybrid photographic space, staging a negotiation between presence and absence through the juxtaposition of different temporalities in the photographs.

Notes

1 I stay with Khemka and Kokiloo's description of their project as "family portrait" (Khemka 2021) in contradistinction with the generic "family photograph." For the purpose of this chapter, the former refers to posed family photographs taken in studios since *Shared Solitude* appears as a pastiche of that tradition; the latter, in contrast, refers to snapshots or candid photographs taken by family members within domestic settings. The distinction remains in the contingent differences in their appearance, although there are several convergences between them.
2 The term is a repurposing of Christos Lynteris's coinage of "epidemic photography" referring to photojournalistic production of a distinct

cycle of images of suffering and mitigation during the third bubonic plague, which broke out at the end of the nineteenth century. The production of these images, he argues, changed the way that fatalities were covered and led to the identification of the plague as a pandemic—as something that was not confined to indiscriminate, isolated cases/pockets but was pervasive on a global scale (Lynteris, 2020). Similarly, the emergence of images of beleaguered hospitals, empty cities under lockdown, migrant workers swarming train stations, or people expressing solidarity from their balconies from across the world became staples of our news and social media diet during the Covid-19 pandemic exposed the nexus of contiguous events and shared experiences.

3 In his essay "Lapsus Imaginis: The Image in Ruins" (2001), Eduardo Cadava asks this question when confronted with the ruins of the bombarded Holland House Library. Following Walter Benjamin's suggestion that history and time is always already inscribed in the photographic image, Cadava (2001) asks how an account of the circumstances in which the image is produced can be discerned when they are not visible within the image. Cadava's inquiry is relevant to my discussion since the family portrait made during the pandemic does not bear any overt traces of the conditions under which it came to be.

4 Here, I repurpose Ariella Azoullay's argument "to watch" a photograph, and not merely "look" at them, such that one can witness the photographic event as an unfolding present and not an ossified evidence of the past, thereby animating the image with different temporalities.

Bibliography

Appadurai, A. (1997) The Colonial Backdrop. *Afterimage*, 24(5), pp. 4–7. https://doi.org/10.1525/aft.1997.24.5.4

Azoulay, A. (2008) *The Civil Contract of Photography*. New York: Zone Books.

Barthes, R. (1981) *Camera Lucida: Reflections on Photography*. New York: Macmillan.

Bourdieu, P. and Whiteside, S. (1990) *Photography: A Middle-Brow Art*. Cambridge: Polity Press.

Bray, S. (2020) Loved and Lost: Grief in the Time of Coronavirus—A Photo Essay. *The Guardian*. [online] 21 August. Available at: https://www.theguardian.com/artanddesign/2020/aug/21/loved-and-lost-simon-bray-phoO-essay [Accessed 3 Jul. 2024].

Cadava, E. (2001) Lapsus Imaginis: The Image in Ruins. *October*, 96, pp. 35–60. https://doi.org/10.2307/779116

Dou, G.Y. (2021) Toward a Non-Binary Sense of Mobility: Insights from Self-Presentation in Instagram Photography during Covid-19 Pandemic. *Media, Culture & Society*, 43(8), pp. 1395–1413. https://doi.org/10.1177/01634437211008734

Flint, K. (2015) Surround, Background, and the Overlooked. *Victorian Studies*, [online], 57(3), pp. 449–461. Available at: https://muse.jhu.edu/article/594949 [Accessed 3 July 2024].
Garden, W. (2007) Photographic Space and the Indian Portrait Studio. [online] *Double Dialogues*. Available at: https://www.doubledialogues.com/article/photographic-space-and-the-indian-portrait-stulo [Accessed 3 July 2024].
Khemka, A. (2021) Shared Solitude—Alkazi Foundation. [online] Alkazi Foundation. Available at: https://alkazifoundation.org/shared-solitude-by-anita-khemka-imran-kokiloo/ [Accessed 3 Jul. 2024].
Khemka, A. and Kokiloo, I. (2021) Shared Solitude. *ANTYAJAA: Indian Journal of Women and Social Change*, 6(1–2), pp. 127–139. https://doi.org/10.1177/24556327221080267
Luttik, M.L.A., Mahrer-Imhof, R., García-Vivar, C., Brødsgaard, A., Dieperink, K.B., Imhof, L., Østergaard, B., Svavarsdottir, E.K., and Konradsen, H. (2020) The Covid-19 Pandemic: A Family Affair. *Journal of Family Nursing*, 26(2), pp. 87–89.
Lynteris, C. (2020) Photography and Pandemics. [online] *Apollo Magazine*. Available at: https://www.apollo-magazine.com/photography-pandemics/ [Accessed 3 July 2024].
Martikainen, J. and Sakki, I. (2021) How Newspaper Images Position Different Groups of People in Relation to the Covid-19 Pandemic: A Social Representations Approach. *Journal of Community & Applied Social Psychology*, 6(4). https://doi.org/10.1002/casp.2515
Narain, S. (2018) Family Intact: An Experience of being Photographed. *The Trans-Asia Photography Review*, 9(1). Available at: https://quod.lib.umich.edu/t/tap/7977573.0009.106/--family-intact-an-experience-of-being-photographed?rgn=main [Accessed 3 July 2024].
Pinney, C. (1997) *Camera Indica: The Social Life of Indian Photographs*. Chicago: University of Chicago Press.
Pinney, C. (2023) What Time is the Visual? Photography and the History of the Future. *Visual Anthropology Review*, 39(1), pp, 24–56. https://doi.org/10.1111/var.12288
Rose, G. (2003) Family Photographs and Domestic Spacings: A Case Study. *Transactions of the Institute of British Geographers*, 28(1), pp. 5–18. Available at: https://www.jstor.org/stable/3804564 [Accessed 3 July 2024].
Strassler, K. (2010) *Refracted Visions: Popular Photography and National Modernity in Java*. Durham: Duke University Press.
Wolf, W. and Bernhart, W. (2006) *Framing Borders in Literature and Other Media*. Leiden: Brill.

12

LIVED THROUGH COVID-19 PANDEMIC

Understanding Lived Experience through Haryanvi Folk Songs

Vasundhara Gautam

While describing the relationship between experience and experiencer, Sunder Sarukkai asserts that 'lived experiences' do not provide a scope for the experiencer to escape the experience or the context. It creates an unbreakable bond between the experiencer, the context, and the content of the experience (Guru and Sarukkai, 2012, pp. 35–37). The Covid-19 pandemic has affected almost everyone worldwide, and everyone has a different story to narrate about their experiences. For many, the pandemic meant loneliness and isolation because of lockdown and distancing from their loved ones. For others, it was the loss of livelihood, hospital cues, long recoveries, piles of dead bodies, the fight for oxygen cylinders, SOS messages, and so on and so forth.

The pandemic created new ways of working and learning from home. It gave a sharp rise to mental health issues, anxiety, and depression. Everyone had a different version of their reality; everyone had a different lived experience of the pandemic. Avoiding the touch of your loved ones was the new normal in the pandemic.

The constraints on physical proximity paved the proliferation of the virtual, and this chapter attempts to explore Haryanvi folk songs sung by women on digital platforms, in this case, YouTube, during Covid-19 pandemic. Haryanvi folk songs on Covid-19 are a peculiar mix of lived experiences, safety measures, and traditional knowledge systems. The study makes the case that folk songs become a tool in the hands of women to navigate uncharted and unknown territory, while doing so they create a different space for themselves. Through folk songs, women

DOI: 10.4324/9781003590392-17

also investigate the fear and apprehensions that developed as a result of the healthcare system's collapse.

In Haryanvi culture, folk songs hold a special place; one could find a large body of folk songs sung by men and women singers in different spaces. According to Sadhuram Sharda, folk songs are the most important folk form in folk literature/*lok sahitya* to express folk mind (*lok manas*) in a comprehensive manner (Sharda, 2011, pp. VII–X). These folk songs constitute the lived realities of Haryanvi society; almost all songs emerge from the lived experiences of the people, be it the birth songs (*jacha geet*) where the desire for the male child is blatantly observed, and the birth of a female child is mourned, or everyday work songs (*dincharya* geet), where women spend most of their time working throughout the day. In a similar vein, Covid-19 folk songs not only constitute the lived experiences of people surviving the pandemic but also an amalgamation of traditional knowledge and state directives.

This chapter contends that new social media has enabled women to negotiate space for themselves, especially those Haryanvi women who are not part of the entertainment industry. Platforms like Facebook, TikTok, and YouTube played a vital role in doing the same. Women exercise their agency to navigate through the new social media, which could be read as both public and private spaces. I am engaging with folk songs on the topic of Covid-19 (*coronavirus ke geet*) sung by women from Haryana on a digital platform, in this case, YouTube. The folk songs in question are a unique blend of women's lived experiences, government directives, and traditional knowledge, sung in the regional dialect to spread the word about Covid-19. It is not to state that Covid-19 initiated women's participation on social media, but it certainly enthused not just the participation but viewership.

"Lived experience is not about freedom of experience but about the lack of freedom in an experience" (Guru and Sarukkai, 2012, p. 36). Experience can be duplicated but lived experience cannot be created or recreated at one's will, and willingly removing oneself from the situation due to the undesirable outcome is not feasible. It creates an unbreakable bond, which in turn creates an absence of choice in an experience. In the Indian philosophical tradition, Sundar Sarukkai (Guru and Sarukkai, 2012) refers to three words—*anubhava* (in Hindi), *abhigyata* (in Bengali), *pattarivu* (in Tamil). The first word exhibits an inherently close relation with the self, while the next two express an explicit connotation of knowledge in them. Whereas in Western philosophy, experience is devoid or distanced from the experiencer or the self and its knowledge, in Indian philosophy, the self and its knowledge are verily a part of the experience. Lived experience not only involves the subjective self but also forms a significant part of the knowledge system. So, the study of folk songs is not only pedagogic but is also critical to study human behaviour and communication practices.

Living through Covid-19 pandemic was/is one such absence of choice, experienced by the world almost with the same intensity. An experience that is not devoid of the self or its knowledge; an experience that is informed or that went through the adversities of Covid-19. People's experiences were informed by pain, a sense of loss, anxiety, depression, anger, and many other feelings. The challenges were more apparent with the economically weaker sections, differently abled people, people with terminal illnesses, and others.

In December 2019, a cluster of pneumonia cases with an unknown cause were discovered in Wuhan, China (Spiteri et al., 2020). And in January 2020 the world was informed about the coronavirus. A surge in coronavirus cases was seen across the globe, and within a short span of two months the outbreak brought the world to a standstill. Since we did not have much information about the severe acute respiratory syndrome coronavirus 2 (SARS-CoV-2) popularly known as corona or Covid-19, every country applied different strategies to deal with the unprecedented situation at hand. Some of the strategies like maintaining "corona distancing"[1] (An Appeal to the Prime Minister during the Pandemic, 2020) or sanitizing oneself are discussed by women in the folk songs. The fear of the unknown not only caused what psychologists call "death anxiety" (Menzies and Menzies, 2020) but also caused panic in every class about food security and livelihood. Amidst the global crisis, India faced its own set of challenges. On 24 March 2020, the Indian Prime Minister imposed a nationwide lockdown as the death toll rose around the world. India experienced everything from the collapse of the public and private healthcare systems,[2] migrant crisis,[3] and abandonment of dead bodies,[4] to lengthy lines in front of cemeteries and crematoriums[5] but still what followed in 2020 and 2021 was unprecedented.

Folk songs were used in several ways to communicate political[6] messages to spread awareness[7] (UNICEF) among the masses. Lakshmi Subramanian (2020) in her book *Singing Gandhi's India: Music and Sonic Nationalism* advocates the role that music played in the national struggle in India. Vishnu Digambar Paluskar (1872–1931) to Mahatma Gandhi (1869–1948) utilized bhajans, songs, chants, folk songs, that is, the traditional folk media to instil the fervour of nationalism and mass mobilization (Subramanian, 2020, pp. XIV–XVI). Rajendra Chapke and Rekha Bhagat (2006) in their paper titled "Traditional Folk Media: A Potentially Effective Communication Tool in Rural Area" contend that social media in the new age is still a challenge in rural areas due to the network, electricity issues, and the like. But the traditional folk media still plays an important role and is more effective as the lingo and idioms are familiar to the rural populace. However, they suggest caution because not all rural areas can be addressed in the same manner; when employing traditional folk media; it is important to keep in mind dialects, cultures, languages, and the like (p. 132). In another paper, "Blending Traditional Folk Media with Modern Media: A Review," Chapke and Bhagat (2000) suggest the coalition of both, traditional and modern media. Basing their arguments on Shyam Parmar's work on *Traditional Folk Media in India*, they argue that both mediums are very important for different purposes and their blend could effectively bridge the gap in communication. By combining traditional folk media with new social media, a wider audience base could be reached to communicate more effectively (p. 5). The coalition also seeks to protect and advance traditional folk media, which is on the verge of extinction in many cultures. Consequently, new social media emerges as a promoter and protector of culturally rich traditional folk media.

Be it the mass movement at the national level or the dissemination of messages at the rural level, women had a significant role to play in it. But the spaces available to women are limited, especially in Haryana, where their presence is mostly limited to private spaces. Prem Chowdhry writes,

> A ubiquitous sight in rural Haryana is the veiled woman who covers either the whole face or just permits the eyes to show. This sight is somewhat incongruous set against the high visibility of women in Haryana involved in all sorts of work in the fields, working alongside men, from preparing the fields to irrigating and harvesting the crop.
> *(1994, p. 1)*

She argues that the veil, or *ghunghat*, in the case of Haryanvi women is a mere extension of their private space as they are never encountered loitering in public but engaged in labour. According to Chowdhry, the veil played an important part in how patriarchy refurbished itself through time to bar women from entering public spaces. Even in post-Independent India, the veil continued to hold its prominence, especially in rural India without a challenge from the liberal or reformist forces. In a 2017 advertisement that read "*ghunghat ki aan baan, mhare Haryana ki pehchan*" (Gupta, 2017), the Haryana government openly advocated for the veil. The advertisement took pride in the veil as a symbol of Haryana's identity. The veil not only symbolizes respect (*izzat*) or modesty (*sharam*), but it is also a symbol of oppression. It is used against women to constrict not only their movement but the spaces they inhabit.

Women are often referred to as naked (*nangi*) or shameless (*besharam*) if they do not observe the veil in public spaces or even at home in front of the senior members of the household. Consequently, the veil also becomes a symbol of maintaining social hierarchy. Moral policing is implemented to uphold cultural, moral values in order to preserve the dispensation. Members of the community and caste-based panchayats (*khap Panchayats*) both contribute equally to uphold the cultural values. Pooja Vidrohi, in an article on women's presence in pop culture in Haryana, points out the role of *khap panchayats* and their infamous mandates (*farmans*) against women for "restricting their liberty and mobility in public spaces" (Vidrohi, 2021). Although things have become a little relaxed in the past decade, still women are often met with a community backlash or severe consequences when they infringe or transgress. One such example of a person who suffered as a result of being in public is Sapna Choudhary. She had endured criticism and public humiliation to the point that she attempted suicide as a result (Inshorts, 2016). The presence of women in public spaces has increased, especially in the entertainment industry. Though we have a long way to go in the realm of gender parity, the mainstreaming of Haryanvi pop culture might help in eradicating some of the misogynistic ideals from the collective consciousness of society. It is promising to note that more and more women are gaining access to education and employment, amidst the violent masculinity that mandates their restriction to the domestic space. The claim is correct in part. The popular Haryanvi music may dispel some misogynistic beliefs, but the same industry continues to create songs that reiterate/reinforce the existing norms to oppress women. Songs like *Ghunghat Bain* by Ajay Hooda and Ruchika Jangid (Gem Tunes Haryanvi, 2019) and *Ghunghat* by Sapna Choudhary and Naveen Neru (Nav Haryanvi, 2019), not only celebrate *ghunghat* as a symbol of respect and modesty and hence should be administered even with force or violence. The various tenets, and trends of the entertainment industry, continually modify themselves to reflect audience tastes. It is an unreliable source of transformation as far as the grassroot level of change in society is concerned. The process of negotiating space with the age-old patriarchal mindset is a tedious one but at the same time necessary.

The world saw massive growth in the digital platforms industry at the onset of Covid-19. Digital platforms like Zoom, Google Meet, and Microsoft Teams, especially gained prominence during the global pandemic but YouTube was quite popular among people even before it. It is one of the largest platforms to display content. Its content ranges from educational videos, songs, and movies to cooking recipes and many more. Unlike Zoom or Google Meet, YouTube has less scope for active engagement, because of which many women singers preferred YouTube. Irrespective of it or because of it, people spent the majority of their time on YouTube during the lockdown. The availability of cheap data, internet speed, and restrictions on mobility made YouTube one of the most popular digital platforms during the lockdown. The consumption and production of YouTube content increased manifolds. To my surprise, I found several contemporary folk songs addressing urgent and significant issues. Topics like politics, election issues, and even the current Covid-19 problem appeared on the feed. The local populace did not limit themselves to consuming the content but producing it. Active engagement with new social media platforms became an obligation, which resulted in creative memes, reels, and shorts to awareness videos on Covid-19. This chapter engages with the folk songs instilled with the spectrum of emotions ingrained in their lived experiences.

Traditional folk media, in this case folk songs, are often assigned to women and are sung and performed by them in safe spaces. Safe, here, translates into private spaces. Women are subjected to these spaces in the name of customs, traditions, beliefs, and like. New social media provided women with a safe space that is private and public at the same time. Women could create videos at home or in known spaces and then share them on public platforms. One could also take many security/safety measures to avoid unwanted attention as well as hate comments and interactions could be limited to the minimum. Shrutika Kapoor, in her work '"Don't Act Like a Sati Savitri!": Hinglish and Other Impoliteness Strategies in Indian YouTube', argues,

> ... while online communication may or may not be absolutely anonymous, the lessened risk of any real physical harm arising as a consequence of online hostility or impoliteness may be assumed to allow users more freedom to be impolite in online communication than in FTF [face-to-face] communication.
>
> *(Kapoor, 2022)*

The stage performers like Sapna Choudhry, Mamta Sharma[8] and many others bear the brunt of community's hate where they receive constant death and rape threats. Therefore, the coalition of traditional folk media and new social media facilitated women to exercise their agency to navigate their way through. This exploration of digital platforms not only leads one to folk songs on Covid-19 but other cultural expressions also about the Jio phone, Narender Modi, Yogi Adityanath, and many other contemporary subjects. These folk songs are a blend of their feelings, thoughts, and lived experiences that provide them with a unique identity. Folk songs on Covid-19 become even more significant as they are not simple folk songs representing the feelings of Haryanvi women but directions provided by them to the men folk and society. It is a greater challenge in a state that is notorious for adverse sex ratio, missing brides, and honour killings (Ahlawat, 2009, pp. 46–47). In the second folk song, folk song 2, Sukal and Nirmala request people to not make fun of them ("*kade mahra majak udaiyo*") as it indicates a concern of a potential conflict from the society. They are almost apologetic about the directions that they have provided. One could sense the pleading tone in all the folk songs given below.

The first folk song calls upon God and informs him about humans being helpless (*bebas*) and unable to deal with the current predicament. It, if observed closely, resembles poet Pradeep's song *Dekh tere sansar ki halat kya ho gayi bhagwan … kitna badal gaya insaan* from the 1954 film *Nastik* (HD Bollywood Songs, 2022). The structure of many *bhakti* or religious songs is similar to that of the present folk song. A sense of powerlessness and helplessness permeates both songs where man's materialistic pleasure pushes him towards disaster. Invoking God not only gives patience to endure the suffering with courage but also a sense of relief. Rebecca Cacho and Fides del Castillo assert that Filipino youth found faith that provided a sense of respite and enabled them to prevail over challenges in life, especially during Covid-19 (Cacho and del Castillo, 2022, pp. 6–8). Invoking God in Haryanvi folk songs also acts as a protective shield against hate or threats. Instructions are often met with hostility. Jesse Graham and Jonathan Haidt, while discussing the benefits and costs of religion, discuss the social function that religion performs. It not only works on an individual level but also at the societal level (Graham and Haidt, 2010, p. 147). In such a condition, folk songs that invoke God provide a natural shield to the person who is singing it. When the women singers say "*Ghar se bahar kati mat jao, Balak budhyon se samjhaon*" or "*Ishwar ki jyot jagao,*" their instructions were paid attention to. Their request to work as a unit and protect themselves against the unknown fear did not fall on deaf ears and gained them around eight hundred and forty-nine thousand views.[9] The folk song also discusses the origin country of Covid-19 (corona) and how it was spread across the globe. Women singers are aware and concerned about the collapse of the healthcare system as a consequence of the heavy traffic of patients in the hospitals. The system also collapses in the absence of genuine scientific information about the cause of the disease. All schools of medicine were found almost ineffective against the severity of the disease. The fear of the unknown gave rise to the panic situation and hence many took recourse in religion.

The complexities of the pandemic manifested differently for different countries and made it challenging to map data that could provide rapid solutions to the crisis. Financial disparities also contributed to the rise in the death toll and the securing of hospital beds. It was then that the singers Sukal and Nirmala requested people to stay at home and asked them to pray to God for a quick end to this unusual catastrophe. The bleakness of the Covid-19 situation is reflected in the lines "*Jeewange to pher milange, liyo mhari ram ram.*" They serve as a reminder of the transient essence of existence and how insignificant humans are in the face of calamity. Doctors and common people, all fall in the same category as far as the transience of life is concerned. The other folk song invoked the past to deal with the current situation. "*Pehla bir ek naam sunaya o, Jin me apni fauj banayi, Chander bose naam tha re uska, Angreeja te ladi ladai*," the folk song recalls the memory of the illustrious military past of "Bharat" by mentioning Subhash Chandra Bose and his army—an army or "fauj" to fight against the common enemy. Women singers are invoking the memories to appeal to the martial spirit of the people of India, when they say "*Bharat desh Janam se yodha, Tam mat dil me ghabrao.*" The sense of pride will act as an impetus to protect their country on a war footing. Since it is a different kind of war, they encourage people to remain in their villages instead of going elsewhere. They remind the men folk about the old security system, "*Thekre lagana*," wherein the community comes together to protect the village from thieves or dacoits. It could also act as a surveillance system to restrict people's movement (Yadav, 2020). Such systems were enabled in many places,[10] since villages were the breeding ground for Covid-19 as mass migration happened in India.[11]

The folk song also discusses basic sanitizing instructions to wash up before entering, or not to loiter unnecessarily. Women in their conversation with the society suggest the involvement of the local authorities such as the head of the village (*sarpanch*) to make people understand the dire need of the hour. The need for these local systems was significant as the government was falling short of people during Covid-19, especially in the villages. It is only in the extreme case that women suggest the involvement of the Haryana police.

Unlike a war song, the tone of both women mellows down at the end of the second folk song. The immediate change in the tone from confrontational to repentant reflects the apprehensions they have about coming out in public and speaking. Women giving directives in a patriarchal society such as Haryana is a little unheard of, especially in public. The shield of religion/God is not available in this folk song. Their being repentant or apologetic could be seen as a protective cover through which they delve into different concerns of society. Another folk song delves into the pride that Haryana's society takes in their culture.

The third folk song is a mixed bag of all emotions—emotions of pride, pain, anger, helplessness, and like. Throughout the folk song, women hurl abuses at corona like "*beiman*" and "*badmash*," to depict the notorious character of the problem. They criticize corona for terrifying everyone and causing many fatalities as a result. Smita Tiwari Jassal, in her work on folk songs from north India, argues that criticizing is often seen as a vent to women's oppressed existence (Jassal, 2012, pp. 135–139). There is a tradition of *gali* or *gari* songs in Haryana, *sithni* to political songs one could find women dissing. Using terms such as these reflects the distress, they would have been in and venting it out was the only available option in the lockdown. According to Eva Jajonie, a clinical psychotherapist from the American Center for Psychiatry says,

> When suppressed concerns and feelings, such as lack of self-esteem; self-defeating thoughts and behaviors; guilt; and anger, for example, are not treated or dealt with, the person uses insults to unleash anger, to escape dealing with the pain or trauma experienced to exert control and feel powerful.
>
> *(Saraiva, 2011)*

Since Covid-19 brought the whole world to a standstill, these women who did not have any agency in their regular lives felt even more helpless. It was a "double pandemic" (Bettinger-Lopez, Bro, and Nargund, 2020, p. 87), as women not only faced the consequence of the disease but also bore the brunt of domestic violence. Sucharita Maji and others depict a sharp rise in the cases of violence against one's partner during Covid-19 in India (Maji, Bansod, and Singh, 2021, p. 6). Their inability to control the situation and loss that almost everyone faced made them take recourse to abuses. And new social media became the platform, where women negotiated their agency.

Another idea that found centre stage in these folk songs is traditional knowledge—knowledge about life, food, and general conduct, information that found space with the new age nutritionists. Nutritionists are reviving the idea of local and challenging different trends in the market. Rujuta Dewikar,[12] in almost all her works, discusses locally grown food instead of importing anything. Women singers also refer to the same knowledge system of living healthy as their protective shield. A system that they have learned through generations of knowledge. They take pride in the *sattvik* food they consume, be it leafy vegetables or milk products. This is also a comment on how corona came to be. Women consider their simple lifestyle and vegetarian food as a defence against the disease. The folk song ends with a hopeful tone, where their traditional knowledge systems and doctors will come to their rescue. It is neither instructional nor aggressive in its approach and is based on the experiences and feelings of the women singers.

Folk songs are generally sung on almost all occasions. It covers almost all aspects of a person's life, from birth to death. Covid-19 is another stage that is added to the long list of folk songs now. Unlike death songs, Covid-19 folk songs are a mix of many cultural elements and not just distressful. Women not only found a voice through their traditional folk systems, but that got representation through the new social media. The coalition between the two allowed women to express themselves in the Covid-19 times. The coalition is not as simple as it looks because a lot of dynamics went into creating these folk songs in video form on YouTube. For example, videos have women with covered heads with *odhni* or stoles. They are showing their faces on a social media platform. On the one hand, where the state government of Haryana is still promoting *ghunghat* as a symbol of Haryanvi identity, these women are slowly bargaining their way in. Another important aspect that seeks our attention is women using their names in folk songs. Often, it is men who inscribe their names in the *Ragnis* and *Sangs*, not women. Women taking credit for the folk song is another step in that direction. And lastly, under the garb of either *bhajans* or invoking historical figures, women are taking the risk of instructing their society to follow the rules. The instructions and directions are communicated effectively through their folk songs.

This study, through folk songs, has investigated the fear and apprehensions that developed as a result of the healthcare system's collapse. Abuses hurled at Covid-19 as well as invoking God were tools in the hands of women to navigate in an unknown terrain and to deal with their fears. Women were able to navigate their way through relatively new social media, where they were not only making a name for themselves but also encouraging other women folk to be a part of the change that looks far-reaching and holds immense revolutionary potential.

Notes

1 In the letter to the Indian Prime Minister, several scholars discussed the pejorative meaning that the term 'social distancing' implies and that it be changed to Covid distancing. An appeal to the Prime Minister during the Pandemic. (2020). www.epw.in, [online] 55(17). Available at: https://www.epw.in/journal/2020/17/letters/appeal-prime-minister-during-pandemic.html [Accessed 7 May 2023].

2 The paper discusses the shortcomings that India faced while managing the COVID situation. Dhar, R., Pethusamy, K., Jee, B. and Karmakar, S. (2021). Fault Lines in India's Covid-19 Management: Lessons Learned and Future Recommendations. *Risk Management and Healthcare Policy*, 14, pp. 4379–4392. https://doi.org/10.2147/rmhp.s320880.

3 The article discusses the challenges faced by the daily wagers or the migrant workers from different parts of our country. The Wire. (n.d.). How Many Migrant Workers Left Cities during the Covid-19 Lockdown? [online] Available at: https://thewire.in/labour/how-many-migrant-workers-left-cities-during-the-Covid-19-lockdown.

4 The article reports following dead bodies in the Ganges. Reuters. (2021). Bodies of Covid-19 victims among those dumped in India's Ganges-govt document. [online] Available at: https://www.reuters.com/world/india/bodies-Covid-19-victims-among-those-dumped-indias-ganges-govt-document-2021-05-15/.

5 The articles engage with the capacity of cemeteries and long queues in front of them. Jain, P. (2020). Endless queues & funerals, scared staff—Delhi's Covid crisis unravels in chaos at crematoria. [online] *The Print*. Available at: https://theprint.in/india/endless-queues-funerals-scared-staff-delhis-covid-crisis-unravels-in-chaos-at-crematoria/437088/ [Accessed 1 May 2023].

6 Folk Songs Strike a Political Chord. (2012). *The Times of India*. [online] 23 February Available at: https://timesofindia.indiatimes.com/city/lucknow/folk-songs-strike-a-political-chord/articleshow/11999653.cms [Accessed 2 May 2023].

7 www.unicef.org. (n.d.). Using traditional folk songs to tackle fear of vaccines among tribal communities in Rajasthan | UNICEF India. [online] Available at: https://www.unicef.org/india/stories/using-traditional-folk-songs-tackle-fear-vaccines-among-tribal-communities-rajasthan [Accessed 3 April 2023].

8 Sethi, C.K. (2018). Mamta Sharma's Murder is a Grim Reminder That Haryana's Raginis Are Targets of Crime. [online] *The Print*. Available at: https://theprint.in/report/mamta-sharma-murder-a-grim-reminder-that-haryanas-raginis-are-targets-of-crime/30392/ [Accessed 15 May 2023].

9 Recorded on YouTube.

10 Kaweenuttayanon, N., Pattanarattanamolee, R., Sorncha, N. and Nakahara, S. (2021). Community Surveillance of Covid-19 by Village Health Volunteers, Thailand. *Bulletin of the World Health Organization*, 99(5), pp. 393–397. https://doi.org/10.2471/blt.20.274308.

11 Mukhra, R., Krishan, K. and Kanchan, T. (2020). Covid-19 Sets off Mass Migration in India. *Archives of Medical Research*. https://doi.org/10.1016/j.arcmed.2020.06.003.

12 www.rujutadiwekar.com. (n.d.). Rujuta Diwekar. [online] Available at: https://www.rujutadiwekar.com/ [Accessed 15 May 2023].

Bibliography

Ahlawat, N. (2009) Missing Brides in Rural Haryana: A Study of Adverse Sex Ratio, Poverty and Addiction. *Social Change*, 39(1), pp. 46–63. https://doi.org/10.1177/004908570903900103

An Appeal to the Prime Minister during the Pandemic. (2020) *EPW*, [online] 55(17). Available at: https://www.epw.in/journal/2020/17/letters/appeal-prime-minister-during-pandemic.html?0=ip_login_no_cache%3Da0ed2229ef52054be79cdb86b5368e7b [Accessed 15 May 2023].

Beamish, R. (2021) Preaching in the Time of COVID: Finding the Words to Speak of God. *Practical Theology*, 14(1–2), pp. 47–57. https://doi.org/10.1080/1756073x.2020.1869371

Bettinger-Lopez, C., Bro, A. and Nargund, R. (2020) A Double Pandemic: Domestic Violence in the Age of Covid-19. [online] JSTOR. Available at: http://www.jstor.org/stable/resrep29816 [Accessed 29 April 2022].

Cacho, R. and del Castillo, F. (2022) God's Benevolent Love in the Time of Covid-19 Pandemic: Articulations and Experiences of Select Filipino Youth. *Religions*, [online] 13(2), p. 162. https://doi.org/10.3390/rel13020162

Chapke, R. and Bhagat, R. (2000) Blending Traditional Folk Media with Modern Media: A Review. [online] Available at: https://www.researchgate.net/publication/280061251_Blending_Traditional_Folk_Media_with_Modern_Media_A_Review. [Accessed 29 April 2022].

Chapke, R. and Bhagat, R. (2006) Traditional Folk Media: A Potentially Effective Communication Tool in Rural Area. [online] Available at: https://www.researchgate.net/publication/280083486_Traditional_Folk_Media_A_Potentially_Effective_Communication_Tool_in_Rural_Area [Accessed 29 April 2022].

Choudhary, S. (2019) *Ghunghat* [online]. Available at: https://www.youtube.com/results?search_query=Choudhary%2C+Sapna.+(2019).+Gunghat+-+Official+Video+%7C+Naveen+Naru+%7C+Nav+Haryanavi [Accessed 3 April 2023].

Chowdhry, P. (1994) *The Veiled Women*. USA: Oxford University Press.

Graham, J. and Haidt, J. (2010) Beyond Beliefs: Religions Bind Individuals into Moral Communities. *Personality and Social Psychology Review*, 14(1), pp. 140–150. https://doi.org/10.1177/1088868309353415

Gupta, A. (2017) Women in Veil Are Our Pride: Haryana Advert Sparks Row; Govt Denies Endorsing 'Ghoonghat'. [online] www.indiatvnews.com. Available at: https://www.indiatvnews.com/news/india-women-in-veil-are-our-pride-haryana-advert-sparks-row-govt-denies-endorsing-ghoonghat-388469 [Accessed 3 April 2023].

Guru, G. and Sarukkai, S. (2012) *The Cracked Mirror*. India: Oxford University Press.

Halat – HD. (n.d.) वीडियो सोंग - कवि प्रदीप. [online] Available at: https://www.youtube.com/watch?v=N_AfVACsjgM [Accessed 11 December 2022].

Haryanavi Geet. (2020a) कोरोना वायरस पर गीत corona virus geet. [online] Available at: https://www.youtube.com/watch?v=nUWEBZvEzAs [Accessed 11 December 2022].

Haryanavi Geet. (2020b) कोरोना का एक और गीत corona ka 2nd geet. [online] Available at: https://www.youtube.com/watch?v=qrr-A7_Fl_E [Accessed 11 December 2022].

Haryanvi Geet Bhajan. (2020) हे कोरोना बेईमान तेरा भारत म के काम /Haryanvi geet bhajan |. [online] Available at: https://www.youtube.com/watch?v=3vwQHFTiNQY [Accessed 11 December 2022].

HD Bollywood Songs. (2020) देख तेरे संसार की हालत क्या हो गई भगवान *Dekh Tere Sansaar ki*. https://www.youtube.com/watch?v=N_AfVACsjgM

Hooda, A. and Jangid, R. (2019) Ghunghat Bain [online] Available at: https://www.youtube.com/results?search_query=Ajay+Hooda%2C+Ruchika+Jangid+(2019)+Ghunghat+Bain%2C+Gem+Tunes+Haryanvi. [Accessed 3 April 2023].

Inshorts – Stay Informed. (n.d.) Haryanvi Singer Sapna Choudhary Attempts Suicide. [online] Available at: https://inshorts.com/en/news/haryanvi-singer-sapna-choudhary-attempts-suicide-147081265891 [Accessed 10 May 2023].

Jassal, S.T. (2012) *Unearthing Gender: Folksongs of North India*. Durham: Duke University Press.

Kapoor, S. (2022) 'Don't Act Like a Sati Savitri!': Impoliteness in Indian YouTube Comments. *Journal of Pragmatics*, 189, pp. 4–16. https://doi.org/10.1016/j.pragma.2021.12.009

Maji, S., Bansod, S. and Singh, T. (2021) Domestic Violence during COVID-19 Pandemic: The Case for Indian Women. *Journal of Community & Applied Social Psychology*, 32(3). https://doi.org/10.1002/casp.2501

Menzies, R.E. and Menzies, R.G. (2020) Death Anxiety in the Time of Covid-19: Theoretical Explanations and Clinical Implications. *Cognitive Behaviour Therapist* [online], 13(19). https://doi.org/10.1017/S1754470X20000215

Saraiva, M. (2011) The Psychology Behind Dissing. *Gulf News* [online] Available at: https://gulfnews.com/lifestyle/the-psychology-behind-dissing-1.858618

Sharda, S. (2011) *Haryana ke Lokgeet*. Haryana: Haryana Granth Academy.

Spiteri, G., et al. (2020) First Cases of Coronavirus Disease 2019 (Covid-19) in the WHO European Region, 24 January to 21 February 2020. *Eurosurveillance*, [online] 25(9). https://doi.org/10.2807/1560-7917.ES.2020.25.9.2000178

Subramanian, L. (2020) *Singing Gandhi's India: Music and Sonic Nationalism*. New Delhi: Lotus Collection/Roli Books.

Vidrohi, P. (2021) Women In Haryanvi Pop Culture: We Must Employ The Gender Lens To Address Double Standards. [online] *Feminism in India*. Available at: https://feminisminindia.com/2021/11/19/women-in-haryanvi-pop-culture-ragni-sexim/ [Accessed 10 May 2023].
Yadav, J. (2020) To Stop Entry of 'Corona Carriers' from Delhi, Haryana Digs Up Roads After Sealing Borders. [online] *The Print*. Available at: https://theprint.in/india/to-stop-entry-of-corona-carriers-from-delhi-haryana-digs-up-roads-after-sealing-borders/412614/ [Accessed 15 May 2023].

Appendix

Folk Song 1	Folk Song 1
Title: *Corona Virus Pe Geet*	Song on CoronaVirus
Dekh mere Bhagwan kaise bebas hain insan	See my God, how powerless is man
Pehla corona aaya cheen me	Earlier corona came to China
Phir inhe bhari udan, kaise bebas hai insan	Then it took flight, how powerless is man
Dekh mere Bhagwan kuch na kar pya raha insan	See my God, he is not able to do anything
Phir failya yo desh videsh	Then it spread across country abroad
Jaise phire tufan, kaise bebas hain insan	Like a storm, how powerless is man
Dekh mere Bhagwan kuch na kar pya raha insan	See my God, he is not able to do anything
Maut ki ginti badhan lag gi	Count of death is increasing
Mach rahya kohram, kaise bebas hai insan	Chaos everywhere, how powerless is man
Dekh mere Bhagwan kuch na kar pya raha insan	See my God, he is not able to do anything
Vaid daktar fail hog aye	Vaidya and doctors have failed
Ho gaya fail plan, kaise bebas hai insan	All the plans have failed, how powerless is man
Dekh mere Bhagwan kuch na kar pya raha insan	See my God, he is not able to do anything
Paise dhela kaam na aa raha	Money is of no use
Reh gaye khade makan, kaise bebas hai insan	Houses remained standing, how powerless is man
Je bhano tum bachna chaho	Sisters if you want to live
Je bhaiyo tum jeena chaho	Brothers if you want to live
Ghar se bahar kati mat jao	Do not come out of your house
Balak budhyon se samjhaon	Make children and elderly understand
Kar do ek Ehsan, kaise bebas hai insan	Please oblige us, how powerless is man
Dekh mere Bhagwan kuch na kar pya raha insan	See my God, he is not able to do anything

Folk Song 1	**Folk Song 1**
Title: ***Corona Virus Pe Geet***	**Song on CoronaVirus**
Dono bakhat dua manao	Pray both times
Ishwar ki jyot jagao	Invoke God in you
Corona virus dur bhagao	Dash out corona virus
Mer kare Bhagwan	May God bless
Ek din tal ja yo tufan	One day this storm will pass
Dekh mere Bhagwan kuch na kar pya raha insan	See my God, he is not able to do anything
Sukal aur Nirmala gavein	Sukal and Nirmala are singing
Apna aur thara dil behlawe	Amusing ourselves and you
Jewange te pher milange	We will meet if we live
Liyo mhari ram ram, Kaise bebas hai insan	Take our salutation, how powerless is man
Dekh mere Bhagwan kuch na kar pya raha insan	See my God, he is not able to do anything

Folk Song 2	**Folk Song 2**
Title: ***Corona Virus ka ek aur Geet***	**One more Song on CoronaVirus**
Bhai re je jeena chaho, gaaman me thekri lao	Brothers if you want to live, patrol in the villages
Bharat desh janam se yodha	India our country is warrior by birth
Tam mat dil me ghabrao	Do not fear in your hearts
Bahu aur bete baalak budhe	Daughter-in-law and sons, children, elderly
Sab mil ke sath nibhao	Get along with everyone
Bhai re je jeena chaho, gaaman me thekri lao	Brothers if you want to live, patrol in the villages
Pehla bir ek naam sunaya o	Earlier brother we have heard of a name
Jin me apni fauj banayi	Who made his own army
Chander bose naam tha re uska	His name was Chander Bose (Subhash Chandra Bose)
Angreeja te ladi ladai	They fought with the British
Bhai re ek fauj banao, yodha ka dharam nibhao	Brothers, make an army, fulfil the duty of a warrior
Bhai re je jeena chaho, gaaman me thekri lao	Brothers if you want to live, patrol in the villages
Sehra me te police phire se	Police is patrolling in the cities
Gaaman me fauj banao	Make an army in villages

Folk Song 2	Folk Song 2
Title: *Corona Virus ka ek aur Geet*	**One more Song on CoronaVirus**
Gorment ki ke baant dekh rahe, tum apni re duty lao	Why wait for the government, assign yourself duties
Sarpanch ne bhi mere bir bulwao	Brothers call the Sarpanch also
Pher sanhi baith samjho	Make him understand in front of you
Tv dekhe te kaam na chalya	Nothing will happen if you only watch TV
Apne hathiyar banao	Pick up your weapons
Bhai re je jeena chaho, gaaman me thekri lao	Brothers if you want to live, patrol in the villages
Ek kehan mera aur pugao	Listen to me one more time
Bekaame bahar na jao	Don't go out without any work
Jo bhi bahar se ghar par aao	Whoever comes home from outside
Saban se hath muh dhyo	Make them wash up with soap
Bhai re je jeena chaho, gaaman me thekri lao	Brothers if you want to live, patrol in the villages
Seema upper tambu lao	Make tents near border
Ude apni fauj bathao	Make your army sit there
Char chale ja char re aaja	Four people go and four people come
Neu duty sahi nibhao	Perform your duty this way
Do sigh jeeli dhore rakho	Keep two teeth fork with you
Hathiyar pehlede thao	Pick up old weapons
Bhai re je jeena chaho, gaaman me thekri lao	Brothers if you want to live, patrol in the villages
Jo koi banda aawe bahar te	Whoever comes from outside
Unhe ude batha samjhao	Make him sit there and make him understand
Kahe sune ki na mane to	If he does not listen to you then
Haryana police bulao	Call Haryana police
Bhai re je jeena chaho, gaaman me thekri lao	Brothers if you want to live, patrol in the villages
Sukal aur Nirmala gaawe	Sukal and Nirmala are singing
Chanel pe baith samjhawe	Making you understand through channel
Bhai re kuch dhayn lagao	Brother pay attention
Kade mahra majak banao	Please don't make fun of us
Corona ne dur bhagao	Dash out Corona from here
Tam mil k sath nibhao	Come together and handle it
Bhai re je jeena chaho, gaaman me thekri lao	Brothers if you want to live, patrol in the villages
Bhai re kade phir pichtao, gaaman me thekri lao	Brother, if you regret later, patrol in the villages

Folk Song 3	Folk Song 3
Title: ***Re Corona Re Corona Beimaan, Tera Ae Bharat Me Ke Kaam***	**Unreliable corona why are you here in India**
Re corona re corona beimaan, tera ae bharat me ke kaam	Unreliable Corona why are you Cohere in India
Tu chalya ja badmash, tera ae bharat me ke kaam	Run away you scoundrel, why are you here in India
Tene duniya saari darai re	You scared the whole world
Ye mar gaye log lugai re	Men and women both died
Re corona re corona beimaan, tera ae bharat me ke kaam	Unreliable Corona why are you here in India
Tu chalya ja badmash, tera ae bharat me ke kaam	Run away you scoundrel, why are you here in India
Re hum saag aur sabji khaye	We eat leafy vegetable
Re hum tazzi lassi peyin	We drink fresh curd
Re hum baajre ki roti khawe re	We eat millet bread
Shirsham ka saag banawe re	We make spinach vegetable
Re corona re corona beimaan, tera ae bharat me ke kaam	Unreliable Corona why are you here in India
Tu chalya ja badmash, tera ae bharat me ke kaam	Run away you scoundrel, why are you here in India
Re ye gau hamari mata re	We pray to the cow
Hum dudh piwein se taza re	We drink fresh milk
Ye hamare aangan ki sobha re	This is the beauty of our yard
Saare pashuyon se naam nirala re	It is unique in all animals
Re corona re corona beimaan, tera ae bharat me ke kaam	Unreliable Corona why are you here in India
Tu chalya ja badmash, tera ae bharat me ke kaam	Run away you scoundrel, why are you here in India
Maahre daktar bade mahan re	Our doctors are great
Tere tukde kare hazar re	Will cut you down into thousand pieces
Re corona re corona beimaan, tera ae bharat me ke kaam	Unreliable Corona why are you here in India
Tu chalya ja badmash, tera ae bharat me ke kaam	Run away you scoundrel, why are you here in India
Tam sun lo re log lugaiyon re	Listen men and women
Pardushan saare le lo re	Remove the pollution
Re corona re corona beimaan, tera ae bharat me ke kaam	Unreliable Corona why are you here in India
Tu chalya ja badmash, tera ae bharat me ke kaam	Run away you scoundrel, why are you here in India
Deshan me desh hariyana re	Haryana is the best in all countries
Mahare dudh dahi ka khana re	We consume milk and curd

Folk Song 3	Folk Song 3
Title: ***Re Corona Re Corona Beimaan, Tera Ae Bharat Me Ke Kaam***	**Unreliable corona why are you here in India**
Re corona re corona beimaan, tera ae bharat me ke kaam *Tu chalya ja badmash, tera ae bharat me ke kaam*	Unreliable Corona why are you here in India Run away you scoundrel, why are you here in India

INDEX

Pages in *italics* refer to figures, and pages followed by n refer to notes.